SPANISH TERMINOLOGY *for* CHIROPRACTIC CARE

TERMINOLOGÍA EN ESPAÑOL *para* EL CUIDADO QUIROPRÁCTICO

SPANISH TERMINOLOGY *for* CHIROPRACTIC CARE

TERMINOLOGÍA EN ESPAÑOL *para* EL CUIDADO QUIROPRÁCTICO

P. Thomas Davis, MUP, DC
Thomas Bergmann, DC
Assisted by Barry Taylor, DC

Reviewed by
Kirsten Addison, DC
Spanish Village Weekend Dean
Concordia Language Villages

ELSEVIER
MOSBY

ELSEVIER
MOSBY

11830 Westline Industrial Drive
St. Louis, Missouri 63146

SPANISH TERMINOLOGY FOR CHIROPRACTIC CARE **0-323-02525-0**

NOTICE

Chiropractic care is an ever-changing field. Standard safety precautions must be followed, but as new research and clinical experience broaden our knowledge, changes in treatment and drug therapy may become necessary or appropriate. Readers are advised to check the most current product information provided by the manufacturer of each drug to be administered to verify the recommended dose, the method and duration of administration, and contraindications. It is the responsibility of the licensed prescriber, relying on experience and knowledge of the patient, to determine dosages and the best treatment for each individual patient. Neither the publisher nor the author assumes any liability for any injury and/or damage to persons or property arising from this publication.

International Standard Book Number 0-323-02525-0

Publishing Director: Linda Duncan
Editor: Kathy Falk
Managing Editor: Christie Hart
Publishing Services Manager: Linda McKinley
Senior Project Manager: Julie Eddy
Designer: Jyotika Shroff

Printed in the United States of America

Last digit is the print number: 9 8 7 6 5 4 3 2 1

Contents

HOW TO USE THIS BOOK

Hispanic is a term used to identify people who speak the Spanish language and have Cuban, Central or South American, Mexican, or Puerto Rican backgrounds. The largest Hispanic populations in the United States reside in Arizona, California, Colorado, Florida, New Mexico, New York, and Texas. Since it is not possible to detail every conceivable vocabulary preference, this book uses a universally accepted dialect. However, you will probably still encounter some Spanish words unique to your area.

ORGANIZATION

This book is organized in three parts and follows a logical sequence of how a practitioner would interact with a patient from initial greeting to specialty appointments.

The book addresses the use of the formal "you" (usted) in situations among adults, and the appropriate use of the informal "you" (tú) in situations in which adults are addressing children.

In cases where two or more words or phrases are appropriate, each is separated by a slash (/).

In this example, the word translator or interpreter can be used to complete the sentence:

I need a (translator/interpreter)—wait a minute.
Necesito un (traductor/intérprete)—espere un minuto.

In cases where several words or phrases are appropriate, choices have been placed into boxes. These choices may pertain to more than one sentence in the section. In this example, any of the choices in the box may be correct.

What is the relationship of the subscriber to you?

Throughout the text, boxes containing helpful information relating to a topic will appear for readers to reference.

RESOURCES

We have included several resources that you may find helpful as you learn to communicate in Spanish.

A mini CD-ROM provides the English to Spanish translation of every phrase in the book. English phrases are spoken by an American elocutionist, whereas a Latin American elocutionist provides the Spanish phrases. Every phrase in the book is included. If your computer is set to Autorun, just load the CD-ROM into the drive. The CD-ROM will do the rest. The CD-ROM is compatible with both PC and Mac, but note that a tray-loading CD-ROM drive is required.

Inside the book, we have included helpful information about the use of accents, verbs, nouns, and adjectives within the Spanish language. A pronunciation guide is also included. At the back of the book, an extensive English to Spanish glossary is provided for quick reference. The glossary is divided into categories such as dental terms, numbers, months of the year, etc. An alphabetical Spanish to English listing of each of the vocabulary words and a list of informal expressions used in conversation is also provided.

Accents*

Acentos

The acute accent is the only mark of its kind in Spanish. It is a small oblique line **(á)** that is drawn from right to left and specifies a syllable that has a stronger sound when pronouncing it. Accents are used generally to distinguish words written alike and identical in form with other parts of speech, but with a different meaning. For example: **papá** (father), **papa** (vegetable); **monté** (mounted), **monte** (large hill). Accents are sometimes omitted from capital letters.

El acento es la mayor intensidad con que se marca determinada sílaba al pronunciar una palabra. Es una rayita oblicua (á) que se escribe de derecha a izquierda y se coloca en ciertos casos sobre la vocal de la sílaba en que se carga la pronunciación. En español es muy necesario acentuar las palabras para darles el significado correcto que llevan. Por ejemplo: papá (padre), papa (vegetal); monté (verbo), monte (terreno elevado).

I love	yo amo (yoh ah-moh)
he loved	él amó (ehl ah-moh)
the owner	el dueño/amo (ehl doo-eh-nyoh/ah-moh)
road	el camino (ehl kah-mee-noh)
he walked	él caminó (ehl kah-mee-noh)
copper	cobre (koh-breh)
I charged	yo cobré (yoh koh-breh)
volumes	volúmenes (boh-loo-meh-nehs)

*From Joyce EV, Villanueva ME: *Say it in Spanish*, ed 2, Saunders, Philadelphia, 2000.

never	jamás (hah-mahs)
pencil	lápiz (lah-pees)

Gender of Nouns*

Género de los Sustantivos

In Spanish, the gender of a noun corresponds to sex. The name of any male being is masculine; that of a female being is feminine. The grammatical gender of an inanimate object must simply be memorized: a bone **(el hueso)** is masculine, the head **(la cabeza)** is feminine, and so on.

En español, el género de los sustantivos corresponde al sexo. El nombre de un hombre es masculino, el de una mujer es femenino. El género gramatical de un objeto inanimado se debe memorizar: un hueso es masculino, la cabeza es femenina y así sucesivamente.

All Spanish nouns must be masculine or feminine.

The definite article *the* has the following singular and plural forms in Spanish.

el (singular masculine)	la (singular feminine)
los (plural masculine)	las (plural feminine)

The indefinite article *a* or *an* has the following forms in Spanish.

un (singular masculine)	una (singular feminine)
unos (plural masculine)	unas (plural feminine)

Masculine nouns require a masculine article; feminine nouns require a feminine article.

the man	el hombre (ehl ohm-breh)
the woman	la mujer (lah moo-hehr)
the boy	el muchacho (ehl moo-chah-choh)

*From Joyce EV, Villanueva ME: *Say it in Spanish,* ed 2, Saunders, Philadelphia, 2000.

the back	la espalda (lah ehs-pahl-dah)
the friend	el amigo (ehl ah-mee-goh)
a rib	una costilla (oo-nah kohs-tee-yah)
the eye	el ojo (ehl oh-hoh)
a skeleton	un esqueleto (oon ehs-keh-leh-toh)
the clavicle	la clavícula (lah klah-bee-koo-lah)

Nouns ending in -al, -ante, -ador, and -ón are usually masculine.

An important exception is **la mano**. In spite of the ending *o*, *la mano* is feminine.

the hospital	el hospital (ehl ohs-pee-tahl)
the tranquilizer	el tranquilizante (ehl trahn-kee-lee-sahn-teh)
the worker	el trabajador (ehl trah-bah-hah-dohr)
the heart	el corazón (ehl koh-rah-sohn)

The days of the week, months of the year, and the names of languages are masculine.

Wednesday	el miércoles (ehl mee-ehr-koh-lehs)
the month of April	el mes de abril (ehl mehs deh ah-breel)
Spanish	el español (ehl ehs-pah-nyohl)

Nouns ending in -tad, -dad, -ción, -sión, -ez, -ie, -ud, and -umbre are usually feminine.

the dehydration	la deshidratación (lah deh-see-drah-tah-see-ohn)

the habit	la costumbre (lah kohs-toom-breh)
the age	la edad (lah eh-dahd)
the friendship	la amistad (lah ah-mees-tahd)
the series	la serie (lah seh-ree-eh)
the health	la salud (lah sah-lood)

Nouns ending in -e should be memorized with the definite article.

the blood	la sangre (lah sahn-greh)

PLURAL OF NOUNS

A noun ending in a vowel forms the plural by adding **-s**; those ending in a consonant add **-es**.

the physician	el médico (ehl meh-dee-koh)
the physicians	los médicos (lohs meh-dee-kohs)
the doctor	el doctor (ehl dohk-tohr)
the doctors	los doctores (lohs dohk-toh-rehs)

A noun ending in **-z** changes to **-c** and then adds **-es**.

the nose	la nariz (lah nahr-ees)
the noses	las narices (lahs nahr-ee-sehs)

Nouns ending in a stressed vowel form the plural by adding **-es**.

the ruby	el rubí (ehl roo-bee)
the rubies	los rubíes (lohs roo-bee-ehs)

Nouns ending in unstressed **-es** or **-is** are considered to be both singular and plural. Number is expressed by the article.

Thursday	el jueves (ehl hoo-eh-behs)
Thursdays	los jueves (lohs hoo-eh-behs)

SPECIAL USES OF ARTICLES

The definite article is used in Spanish, but omitted in English as follows.

1. Before the names of languages, except after **hablar, en,** or **de:**

Spanish is important.	El español es importante. (Ehl ehs-pah-nyohl ehs eem-pohr-tahn-teh)
My friend speaks French.	Mi amigo habla francés. (Mee ah-mee-goh ah-blah frahn-sehs)
The whole book is in German.	Todo el libro está en alemán. (Toh-doh ehl lee-broh ehs-tah ehn ah-leh-mahn)

2. Before titles, except when addressing the person:

Mr. Gomez left yesterday.	El señor Gómez salió ayer. (Ehl seh-nyohr Goh-mehs sah-lee-oh ah-yehr)
How are you, Mrs. García?	¿Cómo está, señora García? (Koh-moh ehs-tah, seh-nyoh-rah Gahr-see-ah)

The article is omitted before **don**, **doña**, **Santo**, **Santa**, **San**.

3. With parts of the body or personal possessions (e.g., clothing):

He has black hair.	El tiene pelo negro. (Ehl tee-eh-neh peh-loh neh-groh)
Mary has a broken foot.	María tiene el pie quebrado. (Mah-ree-ah tee-eh-neh ehl pee-eh keh-brah-doh)

4. With the time of day (la hora, the hour; las horas, the hours):

It is one o'clock.	Es la una. (Ehs lah oo-nah)
I go to sleep at eleven.	Me duermo a las once. (Meh doo-ehr-moh ah lahs ohn-seh)

5. With the names of seasons:

I like summer.	Me gusta el verano. (Meh goos-tah ehl beh-rah-noh)

6. With the days of the week, except after the verb ser (to be):

I go downtown (on) Tuesdays.	Los martes voy al centro. (Lohs mahr-tehs boy ahl sehn-troh)
Today is Monday.	Hoy es lunes. (Oh-ee ehs loo-nehs)

7. Before certain geographic areas:

Canada	el Canadá (ehl Kah-nah-dah)
Argentina	la Argentina (lah Ahr-hehn-tee-nah)

NEUTER ARTICLE *LO*

1. The neuter article **lo** precedes an adjective used as a noun to express a quality or an abstract idea.

I like red (that which is red).	Me gusta lo rojo. (Meh goos-tah loh roh-hoh)
I think the same as you.	Pienso lo mismo que usted. (Pee-ehn-soh loh mees-moh keh oos-tehd)

2. **Lo** + adjective or adverb + **que** = *how.*

I see how good she is.	Ya veo lo buena que es. (Yah beh-oh loh boo-eh-nah keh ehs)

Since the article **lo** is neuter, it has no plural form. Therefore, **lo** is used whether the adjective is masculine or feminine, singular or plural.

OMISSION OF ARTICLES

1. The definite article is omitted in the following cases.

   A. Before nouns in a position:

   Austin, the capital of Texas, is at the center of the state.

   Austin, capital de Tejas, está en el centro del estado.

   B. Before numerals expressing the numerical order of rulers:

Charles the Fifth	Carlos Quinto (Kahr-lohs Keen-toh)
Mary the Second	María Segunda (Mah-ree-ah Seh-goon-dah)

2. The indefinite article is omitted before predicate nouns denoting a class or group (social class, occupation, nationality, religion, etc.):

He is a barber.	Es barbero. (Ehs bahr-beh-roh)
I am Mexican.	Soy mexicana. (Soh-ee meh-hee-kah-nah)
I want to be a nurse.	Quiero ser enfermera. (Kee-eh-roh sehr ehn-fehr-meh-rah)

If the predicate noun is modified, the indefinite article is stated:

He is a hard-working barber.	Es un barbero muy trabajador. (Ehs oon bahr-beh-roh moo-ee trah-bah-hah-dohr)
I want to be a good nurse.	Quiero ser una buena enfermera. (Kee-eh-roh sehr oo-nah boo-eh-nah ehn-fehr-meh-rah)

Adjectives and Pronouns*

Adjetivos y Pronombres

Adjectives describe nouns and pronouns. In Spanish, adjectives are placed after the noun. They agree in number and gender with the noun they modify.

ADJECTIVES ENDING IN -O

Masculine singular:	The patient is happy. El paciente está contento. (Ehl pah-see-ehn-teh ehs-tah kohn-tehn-toh)
Feminine singular:	She is happy. Ella está contenta. (Eh-yah ehs-tah kohn-tehn-tah)
Masculine plural:	They are happy. Ellos están contentos. (Eh-yohs ehs-tahn kohn-tehn-tohs)
Feminine plural:	They are happy. Ellas están contentas. (Eh-yahs ehs-tahn kohn-tehn-tahs)

ADJECTIVES ENDING IN –E

Masculine singular:	He is sad. Él está triste. (Ehl ehs-tah trees-teh)
Feminine singular:	She is sad. Ella está triste. (Eh-yah ehs-tah trees-teh)

*From Joyce EV, Villanueva ME: *Say it in Spanish,* ed 2, Saunders, Philadelphia, 2000.

Masculine plural:	They are sad. Ellos están tristes. (Eh-yohs ehs-tahn trees-tehs)
Feminine plural:	They are sad. Ellas están tristes. (Eh-yahs ehs-tahn trees-tehs)

ADJECTIVES ENDING IN A CONSONANT

Masculine singular:	The procedure is difficult. El procedimiento es difícil. (Ehl proh-seh-dee-mee-ehn-toh ehs dee-fee-seel)
Feminine singular:	The measurement is difficult. La medida es difícil. (Lah meh-dee-dah ehs dee-fee-seel)
Masculine plural:	The exams are difficult. Los exámenes son difíciles. (Lohs ehx-ah-meh-nehs sohn dee-fee-see-lehs)
Feminine plural:	The measurements are difficult. Las medidas son difíciles. (Lahs meh-dee-dahs sohn dee-fee-see-lehs)

Demonstrative adjectives precede the nouns they modify and agree with them in number and gender.

this book	este libro (ehs-teh lee-broh)
these pens	estas plumas (ehs-tahs ploo-mahs)

Este (*this*) refers to what is near or directly concerns me.

Esos (*those*) refers to what is near or directly concerns you.

Aquel (*that*) refers to what is remote to the speaker or the person addressed.

This pencil is red.	Este lápiz es rojo. (Ehs-teh lah-pees ehs roh-hoh)

John, give me that bone.	Juan, déme aquel hueso. (Hoo-ahn, deh-meh ah-kehl oo-eh-soh)

SOME COMMON LIMITING ADJECTIVES

all, everything	todo (toh-doh)
bad	malo (mah-loh)
better	mejor (meh-hohr)
big (*age*)	grande (grahn-deh)
first	primero (pree-meh-roh)
fourth	cuarto (koo-ahr-toh)
good	bueno (boo-eh-noh)
less	menos (meh-nohs)
little, few	poco (poh-koh)
more	mucho, más (moo-choh, mahs)
nothing	nada (nah-dah)
one, a, an	un (oon)
small (*age, fit*)	pequeño/chico (peh-keh-nyoh/chee-koh)

POSSESSIVE PRONOUNS

	Singular	**Plural**
mine	el mío, la mía (ehl mee-oh, lah mee-ah)	los míos, las mías (lohs mee-ohs, lahs mee-ahs)
yours	el tuyo, la tuya (ehl too-yoh, lah too-yah)	los tuyos, las tuyas (lohs too-yohs, lahs too-yahs)

his, hers, theirs	el suyo, la suya (ehl soo-yoh, lah soo-yah)	los suyos, las suyas (lohs soo-yohs, lahs soo-yahs)
ours	el nuestro, la nuestra (ehl noo-ehs-troh, lah noo-ehs-trah)	los nuestros, las nuestras (lohs noo-ehs-trohs, lahs noo-ehs-trahs)

Possessive pronouns are formed by the definite article + the long form of the possessive adjective.

My nose is prettier than yours.	Mi nariz es más bonita que la tuya. (Mee nah-rees ehs mahs boh-nee-tah keh lah too-yah)

After the verb **ser**, the article preceding the possessive pronoun is generally omitted.

The bones are mine.	Los huesos son míos. (Lohs oo-eh-sohs soh mee-ohs)
That gown is yours.	Aquella bata es tuya. (Ah-keh-yah bah-tah ehs too-yah)
These books are mine.	Estos libros son míos. (Ehs-tohs lee-brohs sohn mee-ohs)

Possession is expressed by **de** + the possessor. This corresponds to 's or s' in English.

his pens and yours	sus plumas y las de usted (soos ploo-mahs ee lahs deh oos-tehd)
Martin's pencil	el lápiz de Martín (ehl lah-pees deh Mahr-teen)
my book and Louisa's	mi libro y el de Luisa (mee lee-broh ee ehl deh Loo-ee-sah)
our patient	nuestro paciente (noo-ehs-troh pah-see-ehn-teh)
her rings	sus anillos (soos ah-nee-yohs)
a friend of theirs	un amigo de ellos (oon ah-mee-goh deh eh-yohs)

WHOSE?

The interrogative pronoun *whose?* is expressed in Spanish by **de quién es?**

Whose pen is it?	¿De quién es la pluma? (Deh kee-ehn ehs lah ploo-mah)
It belongs to the doctor.	Es del doctor. (Ehs dehl dohk-tohr)
Whose card is it?	¿De quién es la tarjeta? (Deh kee-ehn ehs lah tahr-heh-tah)
Mr. García's.	Del señor García. (Dehl seh-nyohr Gahr-see-ah)
Whose X-rays are these?	¿De quién son estas radiografías? (Deh kee-ehn sohn ehs-tahs rah-dee-oh-grah-fee-ahs)
They are Mrs. Luna's.	Son de la señora Luna. (Sohn deh lah seh-nyoh-rah Loo-nah)

SOME COMMON PREPOSITIONS

about	acerca de (ah-sehr-kah deh)
according	según (seh-goon)
after	después de (dehs-poo-ehs deh)
against	contra (kohn-trah)
among, between	entre (ehn-treh)
around	alrededor de (ahl-reh-deh-dohr deh)
before	antes de (ahn-tehs deh)
behind	detrás de (deh-trahs deh)

beneath, under	debajo de (deh-bah-hoh deh)
beside	además de (ah-deh-mahs deh)
during	durante (doo-rahn-teh)
far	lejos de (leh-hohs deh)
for	para (pah-rah)
for, by, therefore	por (pohr)
from, of	de (deh)
in, or	en (ehn)
in front of	enfrente de (ehn-frehn-teh deh)
in front of	delante de (deh-lahn-teh deh)
near	cerca de (sehr-kah deh)
outside of	fuera de (foo-eh-rah deh)
over, above	sobre (soh-breh)
since	desde (dehs-deh)
to, at	a (ah)
toward	hacia (ah-see-ah)
until	hasta (ahs-tah)
with	con (kohn)
within	dentro de (dehn-troh deh)

TABLE 1 Feminine and Masculine Adjectives / TABLA 1 Adjetivos femeninos y masculinos

Adjective	Feminine	Masculine
this	esta (ehs-tah)	este (ehs-teh)
these	estas (ehs-tahs)	estos (ehs-tohs)
that	esa (eh-sah)	ese (eh-seh)
those	esas (eh-sahs)	esos (eh-sohs)
that	aquella (ah-keh-yah)	aquel (ah-kehl)
those	aquellas (ah-keh-yahs)	aquellos (ah-keh-yohs)

TABLE 2 Personal Pronouns / TABLA 2 Pronombres personales

Singular	Plural
I yo (yoh)	we (masculine) nosotros (noh-soh-trohs) we (feminine) nosotras (noh-soh-trahs)
you (familiar) tú (too)	you vosotros/as (boh-soh-trohs/ahs)
you (formal) usted (oos-tehd)	you ustedes (oos-teh-dehs)
he él (ehl)	they (masculine) ellos (eh-yohs)
she ella (eh-yah)	they (feminine) ellas (eh-yahs)

Verbs

Verbos

Verbs are to a sentence what the spinal cord is to the body. Verbs give structure to a sentence because they tell us what is being done and when it is being done; for example: I *talk* to the nurse (present), I *talked* to the nurse (past), I *will talk* to the nurse (future).

Los verbos son para una oración lo que la espina dorsal es para el cuerpo. Los verbos dan estructura a una oración al indicar qué es lo que se está haciendo y cuándo se está haciendo; por ejemplo: Yo *hablo* con la enfermera (presente), Yo *hablé* con la enfermera ayer (pasado), Yo *hablaré* con la enfermera mañana (futuro).

Regular verbs end in **-ar, -er,** or **-ir** in Spanish. They are easy to conjugate because you usually take the stem of the verb and add the endings: **o, as, a, amos, an.** See Table 1.

Los verbos regulares tienen la terminación *-ar*, *-er*, o *-ir* en español. Son fáciles de conjugarse ya que usualmente se toma la raíz del verbo y se le agrega la terminación: *o, as, a, amos, -an*. Vea la Tabla 1.

to auscultate	auscultar (ah-oos-kool-tahr)
to be born	nacer (nah-sehr)
to become ill	enfermarse (ehn-fehr-mahr-seh)
to bring near	acercar (ah-sehr-kahr)
to call	llamar (yah-mahr)
to die	morir (moh-reer)
to eat	comer (koh-mehr)

to examine	examinar (ehx-ah-mee-nahr)
to get better	mejorar (meh-hoh-rahr)
to heal	sanar (sah-nahr)
to hear	oír (oh-eer)
to hurt	doler (doh-lehr)
to leave (behind)	dejar (deh-hahr)
to listen	escuchar (ehs-koo-chahr)
to live	vivir (bee-beer)
to name	nombrar (nohm-brahr)
to operate	operar (oh-peh-rahr)
to palpate	palpar (pahl-pahr)
to revise	revisar (reh-bee-sahr)
to see	ver (behr)
to vomit	vomitar (boh-mee-tahr)
to agree	acordar (ah-kohr-dahr)
to bore	aburrir (ah-boo-reer)
to come	venir (beh-neer)
to deserve	merecer (meh-reh-sehr)
to finish	acabar (ah-kah-bahr)
to go out	salir (sah-leer)
to let go	soltar (sohl-tahr)

to need	necesitar (neh-seh-see-tahr)
to reach	alcanzar (ahl-kahn-sahr)
to remain	quedar (keh-dahr)
to stop	parar (pah-rahr)
to take out	sacar (sah-kahr)
to walk	caminar (kah-mee-nahr)

Personal pronouns designate who is performing the action. Many times it is not necessary to include the personal pronouns when conjugating a verb or using it in a sentence.

Los pronombres personales designan a las personas que ejecutan la acción. Muchas veces no es necesario usar el pronombre al conjugar verbos o al usarlos en una oración.

PERSONAL PRONOUNS

I	yo (yoh)
you (*informal*)	tú (too)
he/she/you	él/ella/usted (ehl/eh-yah/oos-tehd)
we	nosotros (noh-soh-trohs)
they/you (*plural*)	ellos/ellas/ustedes (eh-yohs/eh-yahs/oos-teh-dehs)

To Feel	**Sentir (Sehn-Teer)**
I feel	siento (see-ehn-toh)
you feel	sientes (see-ehn-tehs)
he/she feels; you feel	siente (see-ehn-teh)

we feel	sentimos (sehn-tee-mohs)
they feel	sienten (see-ehn-tehn)
To Sit Down	**Sentarse (Sehn-Tahr-Seh)**
I sit	me siento (meh see-ehn-toh)
you sit	te sientas (teh see-ehn-tahs)
he/she sits; you sit	se sienta (seh see-ehn-tah)
we sit	nos sentamos (nohs sehn-tah-mohs)
they sit	se sientan (seh see-ehn-tahn)

The reflexive pronouns change the verb's action.

Los pronombres reflexivos cambian la acción del verbo.

Mover (To Move)

Action On Self	**Action On Object**
yo me muevo (yoh meh moo-eh-boh)	yo muevo (yoh moo-eh-boh)

tú te mueves
(too teh moo-eh-behs)
tú mueves
(too moo-eh-behs)
él/ella se mueve
(ehl/eh-yah seh moo-eh-beh)
él/ella mueve
(ehl/eh-yah moo-eh-beh)
nosotros nos movemos
(noh-soh-trohs nohs moh-beh-mohs)
nosotros movemos
(noh-soh-trohs moh-beh-mohs)
ellos/ellas se mueven
(eh-yohs/eh-yahs seh moo-eh-behn)
ellos/ellas mueven
(eh-yohs/eh-yahs moo-eh-behn)

to advise	aconsejar (ah-kohn-seh-hahr)
to ask	preguntar (preh-goon-tahr)
to bathe	bañar (bah-nyahr)
to be afraid	temer (teh-mehr)
to believe	creer (kreh-ehr)
to boil	hervir (ehr-beer)
to break	romper (rohm-pehr)
to build	construir (kohns-troo-eer)
to carry	llevar (yeh-bahr)
to change	cambiar (kahm-bee-ahr)
to clean	limpiar (leem-pee-ahr)
to communicate	comunicar (koh-moo-nee-kahr)
to complain	quejar (keh-hahr)
to conduct	conducir (kohn-doo-seer)
to confuse	confundir (kohn-foon-deer)
to cook	cocinar (koh-see-nahr)
to cover	cubrir (koo-breer)
to cry	llorar (yoh-rahr)
to cut	cortar (kohr-tahr)
to deny	negar (neh-gahr)
to destroy	destruir (dehs-troo-eer)

to disappear	desaparecer (deh-sah-pah-reh-sehr)
to discover, find	descubrir (dehs-koo-breer)
to do/make	hacer (ah-sehr)
to drink	beber (beh-behr)
to eat breakfast	desayunar (deh-sah-yoo-nahr)
to embrace	abrazar (ah-brah-sahr)
to employ	emplear (ehm-pleh-ahr)
to feel	sentir (sehn-teer)
to fill	llenar (yeh-nahr)
to find	hallar/encontrar (ah-yahr)
to fix	componer/arreglar (kohm-poh-nehr)
to fly	volar (boh-lahr)
to get up, raise	levantar (leh-bahn-tahr)
to give	dar (dahr)
to go	ir (eer)
to go to bed, lie down	acostarse (ah-kohs-tahr-seh)
to have	haber/tener (ah-behr)
to hunt	cazar (kah-sahr)
to joke, kid	bromear (broh-meh-ahr)
to jump	saltar (sahl-tahr)
to kiss	besar (beh-sahr)

to know	conocer (koh-noh-sehr)
to lose	perder (pehr-dehr)
to marry	casar (kah-sahr)
to paint	pintar (peen-tahr)
to point	señalar (seh-nyah-lahr)
to promise	prometer (proh-meh-tehr)
to receive	recibir (reh-see-beer)
to recognize	reconocer (reh-koh-noh-sehr)
to remember	acordar/recordar (ah-kohr-dahr/reh-kohr-dahr)
to respond	responder (rehs-pohn-dehr)
to return	regresar/volver (reh-greh-sahr/bohl-behr)
to scream	gritar (gree-tahr)
to see	ver (behr)
to sell	vender (behn-dehr)
to serve	servir (sehr-beer)
to shake	temblar (tehm-blahr)
to sit	sentar (sehn-tahr)
to sleep	dormir (dohr-meer)
to speak	hablar (ah-blahr)
to start	comenzar (koh-mehn-sahr)
to step	pisar (pee-sahr)

to suffer	sufrir (soo-freer)
to take	tomar (toh-mahr)
to thank for	agradecer (ah-grah-deh-sehr)
to try	tratar (trah-tahr)
to turn	voltear (bohl-teh-ahr)
to turn off	apagar (ah-pah-gahr)
to want	querer (keh-rehr)
to wash	lavar (lah-bahr)
to wish	desear (deh-seh-ahr)
to work	trabajar (trah-bah-hahr)
to accept	aceptar (ah-sehp-tahr)
to activate	activar (ahk-tee-bahr)
to administer	administrar (ahd-mee-nees-trahr)
to authorize	autorizar (ah-oo-toh-ree-sahr)
to beat, knock	golpear (gohl-peh-ahr)
to bleed	sangrar (sahn-grahr)
to conserve	conservar (kohn-sehr-bahr)
to control	controlar (kohn-troh-lahr)
to evaluate	evaluar (eh-bah-loo-ahr)
to hit	pegar (peh-gahr)
to inform	informar (een-fohr-mahr)

to interpret	interpretar (een-tehr-preh-tahr)
to present	presentar (preh-sehn-tahr)
to protect	protejer (proh-teh-hehr)
to provoke	provocar (proh-boh-kahr)
to reduce	reducir (reh-doo-seer)
to revise	revisar (reh-bee-sahr)
to select	seleccionar (seh-lehk-see-oh-nahr)
to separate	separar (seh-pah-rahr)
to suspend	suspender (soos-pehn-dehr)
to write	escribir (ehs-kree-beer)

The verbs **ser** and **estar** both translate in English as *to be*, but they are not interchangeable. Both are irregular in the present and the past tense.

Los verbos *ser* y *estar* se traducen al inglés *to be*, pero no se intercambian. Los dos verbos son irregulares en el tiempo presente y en el pasado.

	SER	**ESTAR**
I am	yo soy (yo soh-ee)	yo estoy (yoh ehs-tohy)
you are	usted es/tú eres (oos-tehd ehs-too eh-rehs)	usted está/tú estás (oos-tehd ehs-tah/too ehs-tahs)
he/she/it is	él/ella/eso es (ehl/eh-yah/eh-soh ehs)	él/ella/eso está (ehl/eh-yah/eh-soh ehs-tah)
we are	nosotros somos (noh-soh-trohs soh-mohs)	nosotros estamos (noh-soh-trohs ehs-tah-mohs)
they are	ellos/ellas son (eh-yohs/eh-yahs sohn)	ellos/ellas están (eh-yohs/eh-yahs ehs-tahn)

USES OF SER

Ser expresses a relatively permanent quality.

age:	You are old.	Usted es viejo.
characteristic:	The snow is cold.	La nieve es fría.
color:	The urine is yellow.	La orina es amarilla.
shape:	The glass is round.	El vaso es redondo.
size:	You are tall.	Usted es alto.
possession:	The pencil is mine.	El lápiz es mío.
wealth:	The man is rich.	El hombre es rico.

Ser is used with predicate nouns, pronouns, or adjectives.

He is a dentist.	Él es dentista
Who am I?	¿Quién soy yo?
We are Protestant.	Nosotros somos protestantes.

Ser indicates material, origin, or ownership.

material:	The needle is metal.	La aguja es de metal.
origin:	The doctor is from Texas.	El doctor es de Tejas.
ownership:	The dentures are mine.	Las dentaduras son mías.

Ser tells time.

It is one o'clock.	Es la una.
It is 10 o'clock.	Son las diez.

USES OF ESTAR

Estar expresses location (permanent and temporary).

Dallas is in Texas.	Dallas está en Tejas.
I am in the room.	Yo estoy en el cuarto.

Estar expresses status of health.

How are you?	¿Cómo está usted?
I am fine.	Estoy bien.
We are sick.	Estamos enfermos.

Estar expresses a temporary characteristic or quality.

He is nervous.	El está nervioso.
I am ready.	Estoy listo.
You are far away.	Usted está lejos.

TABLE 3 Regular Verb | **TABLA 3 Verbo regular**

Verb	Stem	Endings	Persons
To live	viv-	o	yo vivo (yoh bee-boh)
Vivir (*bee-beer*)	viv-	es	tú vives (too bee-behs)
	viv-	e	el/ella vive (ehl/eh-yah bee-beh)
	viv-	*imos*	nosotros vivimos (noh-soh-trohs bee-bee-mohs)
	viv-	en	ellos/ellas viven (eh-yohs/eh-yahs bee-behn)

TABLE 4 Present and Past Tense | **TABLA 4 Tiempo presente y pasado**

VERB: to eat	**comer**	**(koh-mehr)**
Present Tense	***Tiempo presente***	
I eat	yo como	(yoh koh-moh)
you eat	tú comes	(too koh-mehs)
he/she eats	él/ella come	(ehl/eh-yah koh-meh)
we eat	nosotros comemos	(noh-soh-trohs koh-meh-mohs)
they eat	ellos/ellas comen	(eh-yohs/eh-yahs koh-mehn)
Past Tense	***Tiempo pasado***	
I ate	yo comí	(yoh koh-mee)
you ate	tú comiste	(too koh-mees-teh)
he/she ate	él/ella comió	(ehl/eh-yah koh-mee-oh)
we ate	nosotros comimos	(noh-soh-trohs koh-mee-mohs)
they ate	ellos/ellas comieron	(eh-yohs/eh-yahs koh-mee-eh-rohn)

TABLE 5 Verb Tenses / TABLA 5 Tiempo de los verbos

Verb: To speak

Present Tense	*Tiempo presente*	
speak	hablar	(ah-blahr)
I speak	yo hablo	(yoh ah-bloh)
you speak	tú hablas	(too ah-blahs)
he/she speaks	él/ella habla	(ehl/eh-yah ah-blah)
we speak	nosotros hablamos	(noh-soh-trohs ah-blah-mohs)
they speak	ellos/ellas hablan	(eh-yohs/eh-yahs ah-blahn)
Past Tense	***Tiempo pasado***	
I spoke	yo hablé	(yoh ah-bleh)
you spoke	tú hablaste	(too ah-blahs-teh)
he/she spoke	él/ella habló	(ehl/eh-yah ah-bloh)
we spoke	nosotros hablamos	(noh-soh-trohs ah-blah-mohs)
they spoke	ellos/ellas hablaron	(eh-yohs/eh-yahs ah-blah-rohn)
Future Tense	***Tiempo futuro***	
I will speak	yo hablaré	(yoh ah-blah-reh)
you will speak	tú hablarás	(too ah-blah-rahs)
he/she will speak	él/ella hablará	(ehl/eh-yah ah-blah-rah)
we will speak	nosotros hablaremos	(noh-soh-trohs ah-blah-reh-mohs)
they will speak	ellos/ellas hablarán	(eh-yohs/eh-yahs ah-blah-rahn)

Pronunciation*

Pronunciación

A sounds like *a* in *father* and is pronounced like a clipped *ah.*

ayudar	to help
el abdomen	abdomen
la amígdala	tonsil
la cama	bed
la bata	bathrobe

B has the sound of *b* in book when it begins a sentence and when it follows *m* or *n.*

el bol	basin
bañar	to bathe
el brazo	arm
el hombre	man
la boca	mouth

The sound of **B** becomes softened when it is located between vowels.

la cabeza	head
el rebozo	shawl

The Spanish **B** and **V** have the same sound.

C has a hard sound, as in *come* when it occurs before *a, o, u,* or before a consonant.

la cama	bed
la cuna	cradle
el cuello	neck
la cara	face

C before an e or *i* has an s sound.

la medicina	medicine
ciego	blind

*From Chou B: *Practical Spanish in Eyecare,* Butterworth-Heinemann, Boston, 2001.

la receta	prescription
la cintura	waist
el cerebro	brain

CH has the sound of *ch* in child.

el muchacho	boy
chupar	to suck
la noche	night
la chaqueta	jacket
la chica	girl
el chupón	pacifier

D is a hard dental sound at the beginning of a word.

la debilidad	weakness
los dientes	teeth
el doctor	doctor
mandar	to order
el dolor	pain

D has a soft or *th* sound as in *them* between vowels.

el lado	side
el médico	doctor
el dedo	finger
el cuidado	care
el codo	elbow
mojado	wet

E sounds like the English e in the word *eight*.

el pecho	chest
el pelo	hair
la enfermedad	illness
la parte baja de la espalda	lower back
eructar	to belch
el bébe	baby
la espalda	back
el papel	paper
el equilibrio	equilibrium
la mesa	table
estornudar	to sneeze
el estómago	stomach
empujar	to push

F has the same sounds as in English.

la fiebre	fever
frío	cold temperature
la fecha	date on the calendar
fumar	to smoke
flaco	skinny

G before *a, o,* or *u* has a hard sound as in the word *get.*

gordo	fat
las gafas	eyeglasses
el gargajo	phlegm
el gato	cat

G before an e or *i* has a guttural *h* sound as in the German *ach.*

la gente	people
las alergias	allergies
los gemelos	twins

Occasionally a silent *u* will precede the e or *i* to indicate that the **G** is hard, as in *go.*

pagué	I paid
el hormigueo	tingling sensation or "pins and needles"

To keep the *u* sound in the *-gue* or *-gui* combination, a dieresis (¨) is placed over the *u* as in:

la vergüenza	shame
el ungüento	ointment

H is a silent letter.

humano	human
hinchar	to swell
las hormonas	hormones
el hueso	bone
el hígado	liver
el huevo	egg

I is a short sound as in *machine.*

irritable	irritable
la incisión	incision
el instrumento	instrument
incómodo	uncomfortable
mi	my

J sounds like a hard English *h*, a guttural *h* sound as in the German *ach*.

la jeringa	syringe
las orejas	ears
el juanete	bunion
los ojos	eyes
la aguja	needle
trabajar	to work

K was not part of the original Spanish alphabet. It is used only in words and names of foreign origin, where it has the same pronunciation as in English.

el kilo	kilogram
el kilómetro	kilometer

L is the same as in English.

la lengua	tongue
la píldora	pill
el líquido	liquid
las lágrimas	tears
los labios	lips
la luz	light

LL sounds like *y* in the word *yes*.

los tobillos	ankles
llorar	to cry
la cuchillada	gash
las costillas	ribs
las espaldilla	shoulder blade
la mejilla	cheek

M is the same as in English.

morir	to die
las manos	hands
la médula	marrow
el músculo	muscle

N is pronounced like *m* before *b, f, p, m*, and *v*.

enfermo	sick
la enfermera	nurse
un brazo	arm
un viejo	old man
un pulmón	lung

N otherwise sounds the same as in English.

la náusea	nausea
nervioso	nervous
la nariz	nose
nacer	to be born

N has the English sound of *ny* or *ni* as in *canyon* or *onion*.

los riñones	kidneys
el puño	fist
estreñido	constipated
el sueño	dream, sleep
el señor	Mr., the gentleman, sir
la muñeca	wrist

O sounds like the *o* in *born*.

la obesidad	obesity
la oreja	ear
emocional	emotional
el muslo	thigh
no	no
el pelo	hair

O followed by a consonant sounds like the English *o* in *or*.

orinar	to urinate
el ombligo	navel
el órgano	organ

P has the same sound as in English.

la parálisis	paralysis
el pañal	diaper
poco	little, referring to quantity
el paciente	patient
la pulmonía	pneumonia
el papá	dad
puje	bear down

There are several silent **P**s, as in:

la psicología	psychology
la psiquiatra	psychiatrist
la psicoterapia	psychotherapy

Q appears only before *ue* or *ui*. The *u* is always silent, and the **Q** has a *k* sound.

quejar	to complain
tranquilo	tranquil
la quijada	jaw
la izquierda	left
los bronquios	bronchial tubes
el queso	cheese

R is trilled at the beginning of a word.

la roncha	rash
el reumatismo	rheumatism
las rodillas	knees
el resfriado, el resfrío	cold in the nose

R is slightly trilled in the middle of a word.

primo	cousin
la varicela	chicken pox
la hernia	hernia
operar	to operate
la nariz	nose

RR is strongly trilled.

el carro	car
el catarro	cold in the head
el perro	dog

S has the ess sound in English.

la saliva	saliva
toser	to cough
el sarampión	measles
la causa	cause
el sudor	sweat
la sangre	blood
la vista	sight, vision

S before *b, d, g, l, m, n,* and *v* has the z sound as in *toys*.

el asma	asthma
los dientes	teeth
el desgano	loss of appetite

T is similar to English.

el té	tea
tragar	to swallow
las tijeras	scissors
el teléfono	telephone
tranquilo	tranquil
este	this

U sounds like the English *u* in *rule*.

último	last in a series
usar	to use
la unión	union
único	only

V has the same sound as *b* in Spain. In most Latin countries *v* sounds like *v*.

el vértigo	dizziness
vestirse	to get dressed
la verruga	wart
el vientre	belly
aliviarse	to get well

W is not part of the original Spanish alphabet. It is used only in foreign words and names, where it is pronounced as it is in English.

Wáshington

X has the sound of English *x* before a consonant.

explicar	to explain
la extensión	extension
excelente	excellent
el extranjero	foreigner

When it stands between vowels, **X** has a *gs* sound as in *eggs*.

el examen	exam
el oxígeno	oxygen

Y sounds like the English *y* in *yes*.

yo	I
el yodo	iodine
yeso	cast
el yerno	son-in-law

When **Y** follows *n*, it has the sound as the English *j* as in *judge*.

la inyeccíon	injection
inyectar	to inject

When **Y** stands alone, it sounds like the Spanish *i*.

Z always has the *s* sound.

el zumbido	buzzing
embarazada	pregnant
el corazón	heart
izquierdo	left
el brazo	arm
zurdo	left-handed
el zapato	shoe
la matriz	womb

Part 1
Parte 1

General Communication and Administration
Comunicación y Administración General

Chapter 1
Addressing the Patient with Courtesy

Capítulo 1
Dirigirse al Paciente con Cortesía

Box 1-1 Members of the chiropractic team	Cuadro 1-1 Miembros del equipo quiropráctico
Chiropractor	Quiropráctico
Chiropractic assistant	Asistente quiropráctico
Office manager	Gerente de la oficina

GREETING THE PATIENT
SALUDO AL PACIENTE

Hello, good morning/afternoon/evening.
Hola, buenos días/buenas tardes/buenas noches.

Welcome to our office.
Bienvenido(a) a nuestra oficina.

I am the chiropractic assistant. My name is ________.
Yo soy el asistente quiropráctico. Mi nombre es ________.

Is this your first visit to our clinic?
¿Es ésta su primera visita a nuestra clínica?

Do you have an appointment?
¿Usted tiene una cita?

What is your name?
¿Cuál es su nombre?

Please have a seat, and we will be right with you.
Por favor, tome asiento y estaremos con usted en un momento.

Sorry, I do not speak Spanish.
Discúlpeme, yo no hablo español.

Do you speak English?
¿Usted habla inglés?

One moment please; I will get someone who speaks Spanish.
Un momento por favor. Buscaré a alguien que hable español.

UNDERSTANDING THE PATIENT
ENTENDER AL PACIENTE

Do you prefer to speak Spanish or English?
¿Usted prefiere hablar en español o en inglés?

Please repeat what you told me.
Repita lo que me dijo, por favor.

I didn't understand you completely. You told me that ________, correct?
No le entendí completamente. ¿Me dijo que ________, correcto?

I still don't understand you.
Todavía no le entiendo.

I didn't understand anything you said to me.
No entendí nada de lo que me dijo.

My Spanish is limited, so please use (simple/everyday) words.
Mi español es limitado, entonces hábleme con palabras (sencillas/comunes).

Please speak more slowly.
Hable más despacio, por favor.

I'm not familiar with that word.
No conozco esa palabra.

What is the meaning of that word?
¿Qué (significa/quiere decir) esa palabra?

I cannot hear you. Please speak louder.
No puedo oírle. Hable más fuerte, por favor.

I did not say that (to you).
No (le) dije eso.

I need a (translator/interpreter)—wait a minute.
Necesito a un (traductor/intérprete)—espere un minuto.

Is this correct?
¿Es esto correcto?

BIDDING FAREWELL
DESPEDIDA

Thank you very much.
Muchas gracias.

You're welcome. (It was nothing.)
De nada. (No fue nada.)

Don't mention it. (You're welcome.)
No hay de que. (De nada.)

It was a pleasure serving you.
Fue un placer haberle atendido.

You are very kind.
Usted es muy amable.

Very nice meeting you.
Mucho gusto en conocerlo(a).

Same to you.
Igualmente.

See you later.
Hasta luego.

Until next time. (See you soon.)
Hasta la próxima vez. (Hasta pronto.)

Goodbye.
Adiós.

Chapter 2
Speaking to Children

Capítulo 2
Hablar con los Niños

Come with me.
Ven conmigo.

Hold my hand.
Toma mi mano.

How old are you?
¿Cuántos años tienes?

You look so nice today.
Te ves muy lindo(a) hoy.

I like your (dress/shirt/shoes).
Me gusta(n) (tu traje/tu camisa/tus zapatos).

(Climb/jump) onto the table.
(Súbete/brinca) a la mesa.

Let me show you how this table works.
Déjame enseñarte como funciona esta mesa.

The table goes up and down, like this.
La mesa sube y baja, así.

Let me tell you what we will be doing today.
Déjame decirte que estaremos haciendo hoy.

Let me show you how this works.
Déjame mostrarte como esto funciona.

Lie down on the table.
Acuéstate en la mesa.

Lay face down on the table.
Acuéstate boca abajo en la mesa.

Lay face up on the table
Acuéstate boca arriba en la mesa.

These bumps on your back are part of your spine.
Estas protuberancias en la espalda son parte de la espina.

As I gently touch them, tell me if they hurt.
Mientras las toco suavemente, dime si te duelen.

I am going to gently push on this one and it may go pop.
Voy a empujar suavemente sobre ésta y puede producir un chasquido.

The popping sound is just like cracking your knuckles.
El chasquido es igual al sonido al estillar/sonar tus nudillos.

I am going to rub here to make you feel better.
Te voy a frotar aquí para hacerte sentir mejor.

This should make you feel much better.
Esto debería hacerte sentir mucho mejor.

Thank you for being so good.
Gracias por ser tan bueno(a).

Chapter 3
Office Administration

Capítulo 3
Administración de la Oficina

FILLING OUT THE HEALTH QUESTIONNAIRE
LLENAR EL CUESTIONARIO DE SALUD

Good morning/afternoon/evening.
Buenos días/buenas tardes/buenas noches.

Thank you for choosing to come to our office.
Gracias por haber escogido visitar nuestra oficina.

I am the office manager/chiropractic assistant.
Yo soy el gerente de la oficina/asistente quiropráctico.

We need to have you complete some forms regarding your health history.
Necesitamos que complete algunos formularios respecto a su historial de salud.

All the information you provide is confidential.
Toda la información que usted suministra es confidencial.

You can sit here while you fill out the forms.
Puede sentarse aquí, mientras llena los formularios.

When you are finished, please bring the forms back to me.
Cuando termine, tráigame los formularios.

Please let me know if you have any questions.
Por favor, déjeme saber si tiene alguna pregunta.

EVALUATING PATIENT EXPECTATIONS
EVALUAR LAS EXPECTATIVAS DEL PACIENTE

Have you been to a chiropractor before?
¿Ha consultado a un quiropráctico antes?

Yes
Sí

When was your last chiropractic treatment?
¿Cuándo fue su último tratamiento quiropráctico?

What diagnosis did the chiropractor give you?
¿Qué diagnóstico le dió el quiropráctico?

How many treatments did you receive?
¿Cuántos tratamientos recibió?

What treatment did the chiropractor provide?
¿Qué tratamiento le administró el quiropráctico?

Did the treatment help your condition?
¿El tratamiento ayudó a su problema?

No
No

Do you have an understanding of what chiropractors do?
¿Usted entiende qué hacen los quiroprácticos?

What do you want to achieve from treatment here?
¿Usted qué quiere/espera obtener del tratamiento en nuestra oficina?

For example, do you want to reduce symptoms, resume activity, learn how to prevent this condition, or receive an explanation of your condition?
Por ejemplo, ¿usted quiere reducir los síntomas, reanudar las actividades, aprender a como prevenir este problema o recibir una explicación de su problema?

Box 3-1 Possible diagnoses	Cuadro 3-1 Posibles diagnósticos
Subluxation	La subluxación vertebral
Trigger points	Puntos dolorosos
Strain/sprain	Torcedura/dislocar
Whiplash	Latigazo
Degenerative joint/disk disease	Enfermedad degenerativa en la articulación/en el disco
Osteoarthritis	Osteoartritis
Fracture	Fractura

Box 3-2 Possible treatments	Cuadro 3-2 Posibles tratamientos
Adjustments	Ajustes
Trigger point therapy	Terapia en el punto doloroso
Soft tissue massage	Masaje del tejido blando
Acupuncture	Acupuntura
Ultrasound examination	Análisis con ultrasonido
Electrical muscle stimulation	Estimulación eléctrica del músculo
Traction	Tracción
Hot packs	Compresas calientes
Ice packs	Compresas frías

EXPLAINING THE CHIROPRACTIC APPROACH TO HEALTHCARE
EXPLICAR LA METODOLOGÍA QUIROPRÁCTICA PARA EL CUIDADO DE LA SALUD

Chiropractic is a natural method of healthcare.
La quiropráctica es un método natural del cuidado de la salud.

Doctors of chiropractic do not prescribe medications or perform surgeries.
Los doctores quiroprácticos no recetan medicamentos o realizan cirugías.

Chiropractic is a conservative form of healthcare that recognizes the human body's ability to regulate and heal itself.
La quiropráctica es una forma conservadora del cuidado de la salud que reconoce la habilidad del cuerpo humano de curarse y sanarse por sí mismo.

Traditionally, chiropractors have manually adjusted the vertebrae of the spine to reduce nerve interference.
Tradicionalmente, los quiroprácticos han ajustado manualmente las vértebras de la columna para reducir la interferencia de los nervios.

Chiropractic includes many techniques aimed at adjusting the joints/articulations of the spine and the extremities.
La quiropráctica incluye muchas técnicas dirigidas a ajustar las uniones/articulaciones de la columna y de las extremidades.

Chiropractic healthcare may include orthopedic assessment, physical diagnosis, sports injury rehabilitation, therapeutic modalities, and nutritional counseling.
El cuidado de la salud quiropráctico puede incluir evaluación ortopédica, diagnóstico físico, rehabilitación debido a una lesión relacionada con un deporte, modalidades terapéuticas y consejería nutricional.

If you have any questions, please ask.
Si tiene alguna pregunta, siéntase con la libertad de preguntar.

INFORMED CONSENT
CONSENTIMIENTO INFORMADO

It is important for me to inform you of the benefits, as well as the risks, involved in the treatment plan I have developed for you.
Es importante que le informe los beneficios, al igual que los riesgos involucrados en el plan de tratamiento que he desarrollado para usted.

I have tried to explain to you the procedures to be used. Do you understand what I have told you?
He tratado de explicarle el procedimiento que será usado. ¿Usted entiende lo que le he dicho?

Please read this consent form, and if you understand and agree to be treated, sign it as indicated.
Por favor lea este consentimiento informado, y si lo entiende y acepta ser tratado, fírmelo como fue indicado.

Any treatment that has the potential for benefit also has a potential for risk.
Cualquier tratamiento que tiene el potencial de beneficios también tiene un potencial para riesgo.

Do you understand, and is it OK to treat you?
¿Usted entiende, y está bien que lo tratemos?

Because you are a minor, I need the signature of your parent or legal guardian to proceed with treatment.
Debido a que eres menor de edad, necesito la firma de tu padre/madre o guardián legal para proseguir con el tratamiento.

Your consent to treatment is always necessary.
Su consentimiento para el tratamiento es siempre necesario.

DISCUSSING FEES AND HEALTH INSURANCE
DISCUTIR LOS HONORARIOS Y EL SEGURO MÉDICO

Fees
Honorarios

Mr./Mrs./Miss/Ms. ________ the fees for our office are as follows:
Señor/Señora/Señorita ________ los honorarios de nuestra oficina son los siguientes:

Examination $________
Examen $________

Treatment consisting of adjustment/manipulation $________
Tratamiento que consiste de ajuste/manipulación $________

X-ray $________
Radiografía $________

Physical therapy $________
Terapia física $________

Rehabilitation $________
Rehabilitación $________

Exercise education and/or supervision $________
Educación para ejercicios y/o supervisión $________

Other________
Otro $________

There are fees for other services provided, which will be discussed as needed. (See Box 3-3.)
Hay otros honorarios por otros servicios suministrados, los cuales serán discutidos según sean necesarios. (Vea el Cuadro 3-3.)

Box 3-3 Other services that have a fee	Cuadro 3-3 Otros servicios que tienen un honorario
X-rays	Radiografías
Braces/supports	Abrazaderas/apoyos
Nutritional supplements	Suplementos nutricionales
Orthotics	Órtesis
Special testing procedures	Procedimientos para análisis especiales

Health Insurance
Seguro Médico

Are you covered by an insurance plan?
¿Usted está cubierto por un seguro médico?

If so, what company is it?
Si es así, ¿con cuál compañía?

Can I please make a copy of your insurance card?
¿Puedo sacarle una copia a su tarjeta del seguro médico?

I will check to see what your insurance will cover.
Verificaré que cubrirá su seguro médico.

Your insurance does/does not cover your treatment.
Su seguro médico cubre/no cubre su tratamiento.

Our office policy is that you pay for your services today.
La política de nuestra oficina es la de que usted pague por sus servicios de hoy.

Your co-payment is $________.
Su co-pago es $ ________.

If your insurance does not cover your treatment, then how do you wish to pay for it?
¿Si su seguro médico no cubre su tratamiento, entonces cómo desea pagar?

If you pay with cash, then we can arrange for a payment plan.
Si paga en efectivo, entonces podemos arreglar un plan de pago.

Your first visit will be $________.
Su primera visita será $ ________.

A program of care will be $ ________ for ________ visits.
Un programa de cuidado será $ ________ por ________ visitas.

Do you wish to pay with cash, check, or credit card?
¿Usted desea pagar en efectivo, cheque o tarjeta de crédito?

HIPAA (Health Insurance Portability and Accountability Act)
Acto de Responsabilidad y Portabilidad del Seguro Médico

Our office complies with the current Health Insurance Portability and Accountability Act (HIPAA). HIPAA is a series of federal guidelines that help to ensure confidentiality of your healthcare records. This form explains HIPAA; please read and sign it.
Nuestra oficina cumple con el Acto de Responsabilidad y Portabilidad del Seguro Médico (HIPAA siglas en inglés). El Acto de Responsabilidad y Portabilidad del Seguro Médico es una serie de guías federales que ayudan a asegurar la confidencialidad de sus registros del cuidado de la salud. Este formulario explica el Acto de Responsabilidad y Portabilidad del Seguro Médico, por favor léalo y fírmelo.

OFFICE HOURS
HORAS DE OFICINA

Our office hours are ________ to ________ on (days) ________ through (days) ________.
Nuestras horas de oficina son de ________ a ________ de (día) ________ a (día) ________.

Our office is open on (days) ________.
Nuestra oficina está abierta los (días) ________.

Our office is closed on (days) ________.
Nuestra oficina está cerrada los (días) ________.

Do you know where our office is located?
¿Usted sabe dónde está localizada nuestra oficina?

Our office is located at _______. It is near _______ (local streets or landmarks).
Nuestra oficina está localizada en _______. Está cerca de _______ (calle local o monumento).

Our phone number is _______.
Nuestro número de teléfono es _______.

Part 2
Parte 2

Patient Evaluation And Planning Care

Evaluación del Paciente y Planificación del Cuidado

Chapter 4
Taking a Patient History

Capítulo 4
Tomar el Historial del Paciente

HISTORY OF CHIEF COMPLAINT
HISTORIAL DE LA QUEJA PRINCIPAL

I need to ask you some questions about your health history. (See Box 4-1)
Necesito hacerle algunas preguntas acerca de su historial de salud. (Vea el Cuadro 4-1)

Chief complaint
Queja principal

Why did you come in today?
¿Por qué vino hoy?

When did this condition start?
¿Cuándo comenzó esta condición?

Do you know what caused this condition?
¿Usted conoce que causó esta condición?

Has the condition been getting better, worse, or staying the same?
La condición, ¿ha mejorado, empeorado o se ha mantenido igual?

Pain
Dolor

Where do you have pain?
¿Dónde tiene el dolor?

Please show me where you have pain.
Por favor muéstreme dónde tiene el dolor.

Box 4-1 Red flag questions for low back pain	**Cuadro 4-1 Preguntas de alerta para el dolor de espalda baja**
Do you have a history of cancer?	¿Usted tiene antecedentes de cáncer?
Do you have a history of infection?	¿Usted tiene antecedentes de infección?
Does the pain wake you at night?	¿El dolor lo despierta en la noche?
Have you experienced any loss of bowel or bladder control?	¿Usted ha sufrido alguna pérdida del control urinario o intestinal?
Have you experienced any loss of sensation below the waist?	¿Usted ha sufrido alguna pérdida de sensación debajo de la cintura?
Have you noticed any blood in your urine or stool?	¿Usted ha notado sangre en su orina o excremento?

Describe the pain. (See Box 4-2)
Describa el dolor. (Vea el Cuadro 4-2)

Please rate your pain on a scale of 1 to 10, with 10 being the worst pain you have experienced and 1 being minor pain.
Por favor califique su dolor en una escala del 1 al 10, con el 10 para el peor dolor que ha sentido y el 1 para un dolor leve.

Would you describe your pain as mild, moderate, or severe?
¿Usted describiría su dolor como leve, moderado o severo?

Do you experience this pain constantly, hourly, daily, weekly, or monthly?
¿Usted padece de este dolor constantemente, cada hora, diariamente, semanalmente o mensualmente?

Box 4-2 Pain/symptom descriptions	Cuadro 4-2 Descripciones de dolor/síntomas
Sharp	Agudo
Dull	Sordo
Numb	Adormecido
Shooting	Punzante
Burning	Ardiente
Tingling	Hormigueo
Stabbing	Lancinante
Sore	Irritado
Tight	Tenso
Aching	Doloroso
Weakness	Debilidad
Throbbing	Palpitante

What time of day or night is the pain most troublesome?
¿A qué hora del día o de la noche es peor el dolor?

Does the pain radiate/travel?
¿El dolor se extiende?

Please show me where the pain radiates/travels.
Por favor muéstrame por/hacia dónde se extiende el dolor.

What makes the pain worse? (See Box 4-3)
¿Qué empeora el dolor? (Vea el Cuadro 4-3)

What makes the pain better? (See Box 4-3)
¿Qué alivia el dolor? (Vea el Cuadro 4-3)

Associated signs and symptoms
Signos y síntomas asociados

Have you experienced any other symptoms associated with your current condition?
¿Usted ha experimentado cualquier otro síntoma asociado con su condición actual?

Box 4-3 Activities that make pain better or worse	**Cuadro 4-3 Actividades que mejoran o empeoran el dolor**
Standing	Pararse
Sitting	Sentarse
Lying down	Acostarse
Exercise	Ejercitarse
Rest	Descansar
Working	Trabajar
Movement	Movimiento
Lifting	Levantamiento
Bending	Doblarse
Twisting	Torcerse

Please describe these symptoms.
Por favor describa estos síntomas.

Providers of healthcare
Proveedores del cuidado de la salud

Have you seen any other healthcare providers for this condition?
¿Usted ha visitado a otros proveedores del cuidado de la salud para esta condición?

Whom did you see?
¿A quién visitó?

When did you see them?
¿Cuándo los visitó?

What diagnosis was given?
¿Qué diagnóstico le dieron?

What treatment did you receive?
¿Qué tratamiento recibió?

Was the treatment you received helpful?
¿Le ayudó el tratamiento que recibió?

Box 4-4 Providers of healthcare	Cuadro 4-4 Proveedores del cuidado de la salud
Chiropractor	Quiropráctico
Medical doctor	Médico
Neurologist	Neurólogo
Massage therapist	Terapeuta de masajes
Acupuncturist	Acupuntor
Naturopath	Naturópata
Physical therapist	Terapeuta físico

Self-Treatment
Auto-Tratamiento

What have you done to treat your condition?
¿Qué ha hecho para tratar su condición?

Did this treatment relieve your symptoms?
¿Este tratamiento alivió sus síntomas?

History of chief complaint
Historial de la queja principal

Have you had similar symptoms in the past? If so, when?
¿Usted ha tenido síntomas similares en el pasado? Si es así, ¿cuándo?

Box 4-5 Self-Treatment	Cuadro 4-5 Auto-Tratamiento
Nonprescription medications	Medicamentos de venta sin receta
Heat	Calor
Ice	Hielo
Stretching	Estiramiento
Massage	Masaje
Support	Apoyo
Rest	Descanso

Have you ever had pain like this before?
¿Usted ha tenido un dolor como éste antes?

Was the pain you had in the past more or less severe?
El dolor que tuvo en el pasado, ¿fue más o menos severo?

Past injuries to this area
Lesiones pasadas en esta área

Have you had any injuries to your ________? (area of complaint, see Box 4-6)
¿Usted ha tenido alguna lesión en su ________? (área de molestia, vea el Cuadro 4-6)

When did this injury occur?
¿Cuándo ocurrió esta lesión?

Please describe this injury.
Por favor describa esta lesión.

Medications
Medicamentos

Are you taking any medications for this condition?
¿Usted está tomando algún medicamento para esta condición?

Were these medications prescribed by a doctor?
¿Estos medicamentos fueron recetados por un médico?

Are these nonprescription medications?
¿Estos medicamentos son de venta sin receta?

Activities of daily living
Actividades del diario vivir

How has this condition affected your ability to perform daily activities?
¿Cómo esta condición ha afectado su habilidad para llevar a cabo las actividades diarias?

Are you able to work?
¿Puede trabajar?

Are you able to sleep through the night?
¿Puede dormir toda la noche?

Box 4-6 Body systems and possible symptoms	Cuadro 4-6 Sistemas del cuerpo y posibles síntomas
Eyes	***Ojos***
Vision problems	Problemas de visión
Irritation	Irritación
Redness	Enrojecimiento
Burning	Ardor
Nose	***Nariz***
Nose bleeds	Sangrado nasal
Itching	Picazón
Excessive mucus	Mucosidad excesiva
Mouth and throat	***Boca y garganta***
Sores in the mouth	Úlceras en la boca
Sore throat	Dolor de garganta
Problems with your tongue	Problemas con la lengua
Problems with your teeth	Problemas con los dientes
Difficulty swallowing	Dificultad al tragar
Ears	***Oídos***
Hearing problems	Problemas de audición
Itching	Picazón
Drainage from the ears	Descarga de los oídos
Ringing/buzzing	Campaneo/zumbido
Skin	***Piel***
Itching	Picazón
Rash	Erupción
Easy bruising	Magulladuras fáciles
Bleeding	Sangrado
Swelling	Hinchazón
Respiratory tract	***Tracto Respiratorio***
Shortness of breath	Falta de aliento
Wheezing	Jadeo
Cough	Tos

Box 4-6 Body systems and possible symptoms	Cuadro 4-6 Sistemas del cuerpo y posibles síntomas
Sputum	Esputo
Coughing up blood	Toser sangre
Cardiovascular system	***Sistema cardiovascular***
Chest pain	Dolor de pecho
Heart palpitations	Palpitaciones cardiacas
A sensation of pressure in the chest	Sensación de presión en el pecho
Swelling in your ankles/feet	Hinchazón de los tobillos/pies
Chest pain with activity	Dolor de pecho con actividad
Varicose veins	Venas varicosas/varices
Fainting/blacking out	Desmayo/pérdida del conocimiento
Gastrointestinal system	***Sistema gastrointestinal***
Rapid weight loss or gain	Pérdida o aumento de peso súbito
Loss of appetite	Pérdida de apetito
Nausea	Náusea
Vomiting	Vómito
Gas	Gas
Indigestion	Indigestión
Bowel movement problems/changes	Problemas/cambios intestinales
Loss of bowel control	Pérdida del control intestinal
Blood in your stool	Sangre en su excremento
Hemorrhoids	Hemorroides
Excessive thirst	Sed excesiva
Genitourinary system	***Sistema genitourinario***
Pain/burning when you urinate	Dolor/ardor al orinar
More frequent urination than normal	Orinación más frecuente de lo normal
Loss of urination control	Pérdida del control urinario
Blood in your urine	Sangre en su orina

Continued

Box 4-6 Body systems and possible symptoms	Cuadro 4-6 Sistemas del cuerpo y posibles síntomas
Changes in your menses/period	Cambios en su menstruación/periodo
Pregnancy	Embarazo
Problems with your breasts	Problemas con sus senos
Problems with your sexual organs	Problemas con sus órganos sexuales
Nervous	***Nervioso***
Seizures	Convulsiones
Dizziness	Mareos
Shaking in any part of your body	Temblores en cualquier parte de su cuerpo
Weakness in any part of your body	Debilidad en cualquier parte de su cuerpo
Loss of feeling in any part of your body	Pérdida de sensación en cualquier parte de su cuerpo
Numbness/tingling	Adormecimiento/hormigueo
Difficulty moving a part of your body	Dificultad para mover alguna parte de su cuerpo
Loss of balance	Pérdida del equilibrio
Memory loss	Pérdida de memoria
Difficulty concentrating	Dificultad para concentrarse
Musculoskeletal system	***Sistema musculoesquelético***
Pain	Dolor
Stiffness	Rigidez
Weakness	Debilidad
Swelling	Hinchazón
Broken bones	Huesos fracturados

Current status
Estado actual

How do you feel right now?
¿Cómo se siente ahora?

Do you have pain now?
¿Usted tiene dolor ahora?

GENERAL HEALTH HISTORY
HISTORIAL GENERAL DE SALUD

Now I need to ask you some questions about your health in general.
Ahora necesito hacerle algunas preguntas acerca de su salud en general.

Systems review
Revisión de sistemas

I want to ask you some general questions about the systems of your body.
Quiero hacerle algunas preguntas generales acerca de los sistemas de su cuerpo.

Do you have any problems with your ________? (body system from Box 4-6)
¿Usted ha tenido algún problema con su ________? (sistema del cuerpo del Cuadro 4-6)

For example, have you experienced ________? (symptoms from Box 4-6)
Por ejemplo, ¿usted ha padecido de ________? (síntomas del Cuadro 4-6)

What problem?
¿Qué problema?

When did this problem begin?
¿Cuándo comenzó este problema?

Please describe the problem.
Por favor describa el problema.

Prior illness, surgery, accident
Enfermedad, cirugía, accidente en el pasado

Have you previously had any serious illnesses/diseases?
¿Usted ha padecido de alguna enfermedad seria?

Which illness/disease? (See Box 4-7)
¿Cuál enfermedad? (Vea el Cuadro 4-7)

When did you have this illness/disease?
¿Cuándo padeció de esta enfermedad?

Who gave you this diagnosis?
¿Quién le dio el diagnóstico?

Does this illness/disease still give you trouble?
¿Esta enfermedad le sigue dando problemas?

Have you had any surgeries?
¿Usted ha tenido alguna cirugía?

In what area of your body did you have surgery?
¿En qué área del cuerpo tuvo cirugía?

When was the operation(s) performed?
¿Cuándo se llevó (llevaron) a cabo la(s) cirugía(s)?

Have you had any accidents?
¿Usted ha tenido algún accidente?

When did the accident(s) occur?
¿Cuándo ocurrió (ocurrieron) el (los) accidente(s)?

Box 4-7 Common illnesses	Cuadro 4-7 Enfermedades comunes
Arthritis	Artritis
Cancer	Cáncer
High blood pressure	Presión sanguínea alta
Heart disease	Enfermedad cardiaca
Kidney disease	Enfermedad renal
Stroke	Apoplejía
Diabetes	Diabetes
Measles	Rubéola
Ulcer	Úlcera
Tuberculosis	Tuberculosis
Earache	Dolor de oído

Please explain the accident(s).
Por favor explique el (los) accidente(s).

Were you injured in the accident(s)?
¿Se lesionó en el (los) accidentes(s)?

Did you lose consciousness?
¿Usted perdió el conocimiento?

Were you hospitalized?
¿Fue hospitalizado?

Family history
Antecedentes familiares

Do you know of any illnesses that run in your family?
¿Usted conoce de cualquier enfermedad que haya en su familia?

Does anyone in your family have a history of ________? (illness from Box 4-8)
¿Alguien en su familia tiene antecedentes de ________? (enfermedades del Cuadro 4-8)

Is your ________(relative from Box 4-9) still living?
¿Su ________ (pariente del Cuadro 4-9) aún vive?

When did your ________ (relative from Box 4-9) die?
¿Cuándo murió su ________ (pariente del Cuadro 4-9)?

Do you know what caused the death? If so, what was it? ________.
¿Usted conoce cuál fue la causa de muerte? Si la conoce, ¿cuál fue? ________.

What members of your family have had any of these illnesses? (See Box 4-9)
¿Cuáles miembros de su familia han padecido de cualquiera de estas enfermedades? (Vea el Cuadro 4-9)

Psychosocial history
Antecedentes psicosociales

Do you have a history of anxiety or depression?
¿Usted tiene antecedentes de ansiedad o depresión?

Box 4-8 Family illnesses	Cuadro 4-8 Enfermedades familiares
Cancer	Cáncer
Diabetes	Diabetes
Heart problems	Problemas cardiacos
High blood pressure	Presión sanguínea alta
Lung problems	Problemas pulmonares
Kidney disease	Enfermedad renal
Seizure disorder	Convulsiones
Chronic back problems	Problemas crónicos de la espalda
Chronic headaches	Dolores de cabeza crónicos
Arthritis	Artritis
Lupus	Lupus

Box 4-9 Relatives	Cuadro 4-9 Parientes
Mother	Madre
Father	Padre
Grandmother	Abuela
Grandfather	Abuelo
Sister	Hermana
Brother	Hermano
Daughter	Hija
Son	Hijo
Children	Niños
Aunt	Tía
Uncle	Tío
Niece	Sobrina
Nephew	Sobrino
Wife	Esposa
Husband	Esposo

Have you ever consulted with a healthcare professional regarding your mental health?
¿Alguna vez ha consultado con un profesional del cuidado de la salud acerca de su salud mental?

Have you ever taken medications for anxiety or depression?
¿Alguna vez ha tomado medicamentos para la ansiedad o depresión?

Box 4-10 Mental states	**Cuadro 4-10 Estados mentales**
Happy	Feliz
Sad	Triste
Anxious	Ansioso
Depressed	Deprimido
Angry	Enfadado
Confused	Confundido
Worried	Preocupado
Calm	Calmado
Excited	Excitado

How would you describe your current mental state?
¿Cómo describiría su estado mental actual?

Drug/alcohol history
Antecedentes de uso de drogas/alcohol

Have you ever been addicted to any drugs or alcohol?
¿Alguna vez ha estado adicto a drogas o alcohol?

Have you talked to a professional regarding this problem?
¿Usted ha hablado acerca de este problema con un profesional?

Would you like to talk to a professional about this problem?
¿Le gustaría hablar con un profesional acerca de este problema?

Food supplements, caffeine, smoking history
Antecedentes de uso de suplementos alimenticios, cafeína, fumar

Do you use tobacco products?
¿Usted usa productos de tabaco?

How many packs of cigarettes do you smoke each day?
¿Cuántos paquetes de cigarrillos usted fuma cada día?

How many years have you smoked?
¿Por cuántos años ha fumado?

Do you consume caffeinated beverages such as tea, coffee, or soda?
¿Usted consume bebidas con cafeína tales como té, café o soda?

How many cups of coffee or tea/cans of soda do you drink each day?
¿Cuántas tazas de café o té/latas de soda consume cada día?

Do you take any dietary supplements?
¿Usted toma algún suplemento dietético?

What supplements do you take? (See Box 4-11)
¿Qué suplementos usted toma? (Vea el Cuadro 4-11)

How much and how often?
¿Cuántos y cuán frecuente los toma?

Recreational or occupational factors
Factores recreativos u ocupacionales

What is your occupation?
¿Cuál es su profesión/ocupación?

How long have you performed this occupation?
¿Cuánto tiempo lleva en esta profesión?

Is your work physical?
¿Su trabajo es físico?

Box 4-11 Dietary supplements	**Cuadro 4-11 Suplementos dietéticos**
Multivitamin	Multivitaminas
Calcium	Calcio
Amino acids	Aminoácidos
Vitamins B, C, D, E	Vitaminas B, C, D, E
Fish oils	Aceites de pescado
Flax oil	Aceite de lino
Folic acid	Ácido fólico
Glucosamine	Glucosamina
Chondroitin	Condroitina
Protein	Proteína

Does your work make you sore or tired?
¿Su trabajo lo deja lastimado o cansado?

What hobbies do you enjoy?
¿Qué pasatiempos disfruta?

Exercise
Ejercicio

Do you get regular exercise?
¿Usted hace ejercicio regularmente?

Do you exercise daily, weekly, or monthly?
¿Usted se ejercita diariamente, semanalmente o mensualmente?

What type of exercise do you perform? (See Box 4-12)
¿Qué tipo de ejercicio usted hace? (Vea el Cuadro 4-12)

Is this exercise light, moderate, or strenuous?
¿Este ejercicio es leve, moderado o extenuante?

Diet and nutrition
Dieta y nutrición

Please describe your diet.
Por favor describa su dieta.

What foods do you eat most often? (See Box 4-13)
¿Qué alimentos ingiere con más frecuencia? (Vea el Cuadro 4-13)

Box 4-12 Exercise	Cuadro 4-12 Ejercicios
Walking	Caminar
Running	Correr
Bicycling	Montar bicicleta
Aerobics	Aeróbicos
Weight lifting	Levantar pesas
Yoga	Yoga
Soccer	Fútbol
Basketball	Baloncesto
Tennis	Tenis

How many times each week do you eat at a restaurant?
¿Cuántas veces a la semana come usted en un restaurante?

Please describe your typical breakfast/lunch/dinner.
Por favor describa su desayuno/almuerzo/cena típico(a).

Do you snack during the day? Which foods?
¿Usted merienda durante el día? ¿Qué alimentos?

Box 4-13 Diet and nutrition	**Cuadro 4-13 Dieta y nutrición**
Breakfast	Desayuno
Lunch	Almuerzo
Dinner	Cena
To snack	Merendar
To eat	Comer
Protein	Proteína
Meat	Carne
Chicken	Pollo
Pork	Carne de cerdo
Beef	Carne de res
Fish	Pescado
Beans	Frijoles
Vegetable(s)	Vegetal(es)
Fruit	Fruta
Carbohydrate(s)	Carbohidrato(s)
Grain(s)	Grano(s)
Cereal(s)	Cereal(es)
Pasta	Pasta
Bread	Pan
Sugar	Azúcar
Fat	Grasa
Saturated fat	Grasa saturada
Vegetable oil	Aceite vegetal
Olive oil	Aceite de oliva
Canola oil	Aceite de canola
Butter	Mantequilla
Lard	Manteca de cerdo
Water	Agua

Box 4-14 Body parts	Cuadro 4-14 Partes del cuerpo
Head	Cabeza
Hair	Cabello
Face	Cara
Eyes	Ojos
Nose	Nariz
Ears	Orejas
Lips	Labios
Mouth	Boca
Teeth	Dientes
Tongue	Lengua
Forehead	Frente
Chin	Barbilla
Cheek	Mejilla
Jaw	Mandíbula
Neck	Cuello
Throat	Garganta
Upper back	Parte alta de la espalda
Mid-back	Parte media de la espalda
Low back	Parte baja de la espalda
Shoulder	Hombro
Arm	Brazo
Wrist	Muñeca
Hand	Mano
Finger	Dedo
Thumb	Dedo pulgar
Hip	Cadera
Leg	Pierna
Knee	Rodilla
Ankle	Tobillo
Foot	Pie
Toes	Dedo del pie
Chest	Pecho
Breast	Seno
Stomach	Estómago
Waist	Cintura
Groin	Ingle
Vagina	Vagina
Penis	Pene

Box 4-15 Anatomical terms	Cuadro 4-15 Términos anatómicos
Skin	Piel
Bones	Huesos
Muscles	Músculos
Joints	Articulaciones
Skull	Cráneo
Spine	Columna vertebral
Cervical spine	Espina cervical
Thoracic spine	Espina torácica
Lumbar spine	Espina lumbar
Spinal cord	Médula espinal
Vertebrae	Vértebras
Nerves	Nervios
Intervertebral disk	Disco intervertebral
Pelvis	Pelvis
Sacrum	Sacro
Coccyx	Coxis
Vein	Vena
Artery	Arteria
Facet joints	Faceta de las articulaciones
Spinal nerves	Nervios espinales
Anterior/posterior	Anterior/posterior

Box 4-16 Visceral organs	Cuadro 4-16 Órganos viscerales
Brain	Cerebro
Heart	Corazón
Aorta	Aorta
Blood	Sangre
Esophagus	Esófago
Stomach	Estómago
Small Intestine	Intestino delgado
Large Intestine	Intestino grueso
Colon	Colon
Prostate	Próstata
Liver	Hígado
Pancreas	Páncreas
Gallbladder	Vesícula biliar
Kidneys	Riñones
Uterus	Útero

Chapter 5
Patient Evaluation

Capítulo 5
Evaluación del Paciente

EQUIPMENT USED IN EVALUATION/EXAM
EQUIPO USADO EN LA EVALUACIÓN/EXAMINACIÓN

The chiropractor uses the same type of equipment for a general exam as the medical doctor.
El quiropráctico usa el mismo tipo de equipo para un examen general que usa un médico.

For vital signs he/she may use a:
Para los signos vitales él/ella puede usar:

- **thermometer for temperature**
- un termómetro para la temperatura

- **blood pressure cuff for determining blood pressure**
- un baumanómetro para determinar la presión sanguínea

- **stethoscope for listening to the heart or pulse**
- un estetoscopio para escuchar el corazón o el pulso

Other testing equipment used in the exam includes:
Otro equipo para análisis usado en el examen incluye:

- **tuning fork for testing vibration sense**
- un diapasón para examinar el sentido de vibración

- **rubber hammer for testing reflexes**
- un martillo de goma para probar los reflejos

- **temperature-sensing device for use on the back along the spine**
- un aparato detector de temperatura para usarlo a lo largo de la espina

- **oto-ophthalmoscope for looking into the ears, throat, and eyes**
- un oto-oftalmoscopio para mirar en los oídos, la garganta y los ojos

- **standing-measuring device for determining patient's posture**
- un aparato de medición de pie para determinar la postura de un paciente

PHYSICAL EXAMINATION
EXAMEN FÍSICO

I will now perform a complete examination to help find reasons for your problem.
Ahora voy a hacer un examen completo para ayudarle a encontrar las razones de su problema.

I will now do a very specific regional examination to identify your problems.
Ahora voy a hacer un examen regional muy específico para identificar sus problemas.

I need you to put on this gown so that I may examine you.
Necesito que se ponga esta bata para que yo pueda examinarle.

Please put this gown on with the opening in the back.
Por favor póngase esta bata con la abertura hacia atrás.

Remove all of your clothing except your underwear, and put this gown on with the opening in the back.
Quítese toda su ropa, excepto su ropa interior, y póngase esta bata con la abertura hacia atrás.

Some of the procedures may cause pain or may increase your discomfort.
Algunos de los procedimientos pueden causarle dolor o aumentar su molestia.

This will help me to determine what structures are involved.
Esto me ayudará a determinar qué estructuras están afectadas.

Please tell me if anything I do causes you any discomfort or increased pain.
Por favor dígame si algo de lo qué hago le causa molestia o aumenta el dolor.

How tall are you? / What is your height?
¿Cuán alto es usted? / ¿Cuál es su estatura?

What is your weight?
¿Cuál es su peso?

Please step onto the scale.
Por favor párese sobre la báscula.

Please stand still as I measure your height.
Por favor manténgase quieto mientras mido su altura.

VITAL SIGNS
SIGNOS VITALES

I will be taking your ________. (See Box 5-1)
Estaré tomando su ________. (Vea el Cuadro 5-1)

I need to take your ________. (See Box 5-1)
Necesito tomar su ________. (Vea el Cuadro 5-1)

A baseline reading that is not in the normal range may indicate ________. (See Box 5-2)
Una lectura de base que no es normal puede indicar ________. (Vea el Cuadro 5-2)

Box 5-1 Types of health assessment readings	Cuadro 5-1 Tipos de lecturas de la evaluación de la salud
Blood pressure	Presión sanguínea
Pulse	Pulso
Respiration	Respiración
Temperature	Temperatura

Box 5-2 Types of problems that can be detected by an abnormal baseline reading	Cuadro 5-2 Tipos de problemas que pueden detectarse con una lectura basal anormal
Health problems	Problemas de salud
A need for you to see your medical doctor	Necesidad de que visite a su médico
An undiagnosed condition	Una condición sin diagnosticar
A need for further testing	Necesidad de evaluación adicional

Temperature
Temperatura

I will now take your temperature.
Ahora voy a tomar su temperatura.

I need to take your temperature.
Necesito tomar su temperatura.

Open your mouth, and I will place the thermometer under your tongue.
Abra su boca y colocaré el termómetro debajo de su lengua.

I will use a disposable sheath over the thermometer for your protection.
Voy a usar una cubierta desechable sobre el termómetro para su protección.

Hold the thermometer with your lips closed.
Aguante el termómetro con sus labios cerrados.

Don't bite the thermometer.
No muerda el termómetro.

I will be leaving the thermometer in your mouth for 3 minutes.
Voy a dejar el termómetro en su boca por 3 minutos.

Open your mouth, so I can remove the thermometer.
Abra su boca para poder quitarle el termómetro.

I am going to place the thermometer in your ear.
Voy a colocar el termómetro en su oído.

Your temperature today is ________ degrees.
Su temperatura de hoy es de ________ grados.

Your temperature is (high/normal).
Su temperatura está (alta/normal).

A raised temperature can be a sign of infection.
Una temperatura elevada puede ser señal de infección.

Pulse
Pulso

I will now take your pulse.
Ahora voy a tomar su pulso.

I need to take your pulse.
Necesito tomar su pulso.

I need to hold your wrist with the palm down.
Necesito aguantar su muñeca con la palma de la mano hacia abajo.

I need to hold your wrist with the palm up.
Necesito aguantar su muñeca con la palma de la mano hacia arriba.

I will be applying light pressure with my fingers to your wrist.
Voy a aplicar presión leve con mis dedos sobre su muñeca.

Your pulse today is _______ beats per minute.
Su pulso de hoy es _______ latidos por minuto.

Your pulse rate is (high/normal/low).
Su pulso está (alto/normal/bajo).

Respiration
Respiración

Your respiration rate is _______ breaths per minute.
Su ritmo respiratorio es _______ respiraciones por minuto.

Your respiration rate is (high/normal/low).
Su ritmo respiratorio es (alto/normal/bajo).

Blood pressure
Presión sanguínea

I will now take your blood pressure.
Ahora voy a tomar su presión sanguínea.

I need to take your blood pressure.
Necesito tomar su presión sanguínea.

I will need your (left/right) arm supported and the palm of your hand turned up.
Voy a necesitar que su brazo (izquierdo/derecho) esté apoyado y con la palma de la mano hacia arriba.

You need to expose your (left/right) arm fully before I can take your blood pressure.
Usted necesita exponer su brazo (izquierdo/derecho) completamente antes de que pueda tomar su presión sanguínea.

I will place the cuff over your arm to take your blood pressure.
Voy a colocar la abrazadera del baumanómetro sobre su brazo para tomar su presión sanguínea.

I will pump up the cuff so I can take your blood pressure.
Voy a inflar el baumanómetro para poder tomar su presión sanguínea.

You will feel a slight pressure on your arm while I take your blood pressure.
Usted sentirá una presión leve sobre su brazo mientras le tomo la presión sanguínea.

I will place this blood pressure device over your wrist to take a reading automatically.
Voy a colocar este aparato de medición de presión sanguínea sobre su muñeca para tomar una lectura automática.

Your blood pressure reading is ________ over ________.
La lectura de su presión sanguínea es ________ sobre ________.

The top (first) figure is called the systolic pressure, and it represents the heart at work.
El número de arriba (el primer número) se llama la presión sistólica, y representa el corazón en funcionamiento.

The lower (second) figure is called the diastolic pressure, and it represents the heart at rest.
El número de abajo (el segundo número)se llama la presión diastólica, y representa el corazón en descanso.

Your blood pressure today is ________.
Su presión sanguínea hoy es de ________.

You have ________ blood pressure. (See Box 5-3)
Usted tiene la presión sanguínea ________. (Vea el Cuadro 5-3)

Box 5-3 Descriptions of blood pressure readings	Cuadro 5-3 Descripciones de lecturas de presión sanguínea
High	Alta
Higher	Más alta
Increased	Aumentada
Low	Baja
Lower	Más baja
Normal	Normal
Raised	Elevada

OVERALL HEALTH ASSESSMENT
EVALUACIÓN DE SALUD GENERAL

Head and neck region
Región de la cabeza y el cuello

I need to look into your eyes with this instrument.
Necesito examinar dentro de sus ojos con este instrumento.

Please look straight ahead, keeping your eyes focused at a point on the wall.
Por favor mire hacia delante, con sus ojos enfocados en un punto en la pared.

Keeping your head still, follow my finger with your eyes.
Con su cabeza quieta, siga mi dedo con sus ojos.

I need to look into your ears with this instrument.
Necesito examinar dentro de sus oídos con este instrumento.

I need to look into your mouth using this light.
Necesito examinar dentro de su boca usando esta luz.

Please open your mouth.
Por favor abra su boca.

Stick out your tongue. Say "ah."
Saque su lengua. Diga "a".

I need to palpate (feel with my hand) your neck.
Necesito palpar (sentir con mi mano) su cuello.

Swallow.
Trague.

Is there pain here?
¿Tiene dolor ahí?

Cardiovascular (blood/heart)
Cardiovascular (sangre/corazón)

I need to listen to your heart with this instrument.
Necesito escuchar su corazón con este instrumento.

I will listen at four locations on your chest.
Voy a escuchar en cuatro lugares en su pecho.

Lean forward and breathe normally through your nose.
Inclínese hacia delante y respire normalmente por la nariz.

Respiratory (lungs)
Respiratorio (pulmones)

I need to listen to your lungs with this instrument.
Necesito escuchar sus pulmones con este instrumento.

Breathe in and out each time I move the instrument to a new location.
Inhale y exhale cada vez que muevo el instrumento a un nuevo lugar.

Please repeat "99" while I have my hands on your back.
Por favor repita "99" mientras tengo mis manos en su espalda.

Breathe normally while I tap over your back.
Respire normalmente mientras golpeo suavemente su espalda.

Abdominal region
Región abdominal

I need to examine your abdomen.
Necesito examinar su abdomen.

Lie on your back with your knees bent and your feet flat on the table.
Acuéstese sobre su espalda con sus rodillas dobladas y sus pies planos sobre la mesa.

I need to listen to your abdomen with this instrument.
Necesito escuchar su abdomen con este instrumento.

I will tap my hands over your abdomen.
Voy a golpear suavemente con mis manos sobre su abdomen.

I am going to lightly touch the skin over your abdomen.
Voy a tocar suavemente la piel sobre su abdomen.

I am going to push more firmly into your abdomen to assess the organs beneath.
Voy a empujar más firmemente en su abdomen para evaluar los órganos que están debajo.

I am going to push quickly into your abdomen and let go. Does that cause pain? Where is the pain located?
Voy a empujar rápidamente en el abdomen y dejarlo ir. ¿Esto le causa dolor? ¿Dónde está localizado el dolor?

Laboratory testing
Análisis de laboratorio

I am referring you to a clinical laboratory to have a urinalysis.
Voy a enviarlo a un laboratorio clínico para un análisis de orina.

A urinalysis is needed because of ________. (See Box 5-4)
Es necesario un análisis de orina debido a ________. (Vea el Cuadro 5-4)

Box 5-4 Indications for urinalysis	Cuadro 5-4 Indicaciones para un análisis de orina
Pregnancy	Embarazo
Elderly (older than 60 years)	Anciano (mayor de 60 años)
Obesity (to rule out diabetes)	Obesidad (para descartar diabetes)
Use of hepatotoxic (liver) or nephrotoxic (kidney) drugs	Uso de medicamentos hepatóxicos (hígado) o nefrotóxicos (riñones)
Exposure to toxic chemicals at home or work	Exposición a químicos tóxicos en el hogar o trabajo

I need to obtain results of blood tests.
Necesito obtener los resultados de los análisis de sangre.

I am referring you to a clinical laboratory to have your blood drawn.
Voy a referirle a un laboratorio clínico para que le saquen sangre.

These blood tests will be used as a screening mechanism.
Estos análisis de sangre se usarán como un mecanismo de detección.

These blood tests are necessary to rule out other problems.
Estos análisis de sangre son necesarios para descartar otros problemas.

NEUROMUSCULOSKELETAL ASSESSMENT: SPINAL FOCUS
EVALUACIÓN NEUROMUSCULOESQUELÉTICA: ENFOQUE ESPINAL

Please stand still, facing forward, as I evaluate your posture.
Por favor quédese de pie, mirando hacia el frente, mientras evalúo su postura.

Please walk forward, turn around, and come back so that I can evaluate your gait.
Por favor camine hacia delante, vire y regrese para que yo pueda evaluar su andar.

During this part of the examination, I will be testing many of your muscles for strength.
Durante esta parte del examen estaré probando la fuerza de muchos de sus músculos.

When testing muscles, I will place you in the proper position and apply a force, asking you to resist.
Cuando pruebe sus músculos, colocaré a usted en la posición correcta y aplicaré cierta fuerza, pidiéndole que resista.

Many of these tests will attempt to provoke your pain. This will give me information on which bones, joints, and muscles are causing problems for you.
Muchas de estas pruebas intentarán provocarle dolor. Esto me dará información de cuáles huesos, articulaciones y músculos están causándole problemas.

Tell me if anything I do to you hurts and where the pain is exactly.
Dígame si algo de lo que hago le causa dolor y dónde exactamente es el dolor.

Where is your pain?
¿Dónde está su dolor?

Cervical spine
Espina cervical

I need you to move your head in all directions and tell me if you have any pain.
Necesito que mueva su cabeza en todas las direcciones y que me diga si tiene algún dolor.

Tip your head down.
Incline su cabeza hacia abajo.

Tip your head up.
Incline su cabeza hacia arriba.

Turn your head to the right.
Vire su cabeza hacia la derecha.

Turn your head to the left.
Vire su cabeza hacia la izquierda.

Tip your head to the right.
Incline su cabeza hacia la derecha.

Tip your head to the left.
Incline su cabeza hacia la izquierda.

As I do these next tests, tell me whether they make your pain better or worse or cause no change, and tell me the location of any pain that is produced.
Mientras hago estas próximas pruebas, dígame si mejoran, empeoran o no causan cambio en el dolor, y dígame la localización de cualquier dolor que se produzca.

I am going to lift up on your head.
Voy a halar su cabeza hacia arriba.

I am going to push down on your head.
Voy a empujar su cabeza hacia abajo.

I am going to push down on your shoulder.
Voy a empujar sus hombros hacia abajo.

Place your hand on top of your head. Does that relieve the pain?
Coloque su mano sobre su cabeza. ¿Esto le alivia el dolor?

Tip your head back and turn your neck to the (right/left). Does this cause any problem?
Incline su cabeza hacia atrás y vire su cuello hacia la (derecha/izquierda). ¿Esto le causa algún problema?

Does coughing, sneezing, or straining cause any increase in pain?
¿El toser, estornudar o estirarse le aumenta el dolor?

I will now tap your arm muscles with this rubber hammer.
Ahora voy a golpear suavemente sus músculos del brazo con este martillo de goma.

I am going to bend your wrist back quickly.
Voy a doblar su muñeca hacia atrás.

I am going to touch you lightly on your arms. Tell me if there is a difference in sensation from one side to the other.
Voy a tocarlo suavemente en sus brazos. Dígame si hay alguna diferencia en sensación entre un lado y el otro.

I am going to touch your arms with this pin. Tell me if it feels sharp or dull.
Voy a tocar sus brazos con este alfiler. Dígame si se siente afilado o desafilado.

I need to test some arm muscles for strength.
Necesito probar la fuerza de los músculos de su brazo.

Hold your arm out to the side with your elbow bent forward. I am going to push down; resist.
Descanse su brazo a su lado, con el codo doblado hacia delante. Voy a empujarlo hacia abajo; resístase.

Hold your arm out forward with your elbow bent. I am going to pull; resist. I'm going to push; resist.
Saque su brazo hacia delante, con su codo doblado. Voy a halarlo; resístase. Voy a empujarlo; resístase.

Bring your wrists up. I am going to pull down; resist.
Doble su muñeca hacia arriba. Voy a halarla hacia abajo; resístase.

Drop your wrists down. I'm going to pull up; resist.
Doble su muñeca hacia abajo. Voy a empujarla hacia arriba; resístase.

Curl your fingers. I am going to pull them; resist.
Doble sus dedos. Voy a halarlos; resístase.

Spread your fingers apart. I am going to push them together; resist.
Separe sus dedos. Voy a tratar de unirlos; resístase.

With you seated, I am going to evaluate the relationship of each vertebra in your neck.
Con usted sentado, voy a evaluar la relación de cada vértebra en su cuello.

With you lying on your back, I am going to evaluate the relationship of each vertebra in your neck.
Con usted acostado sobre su espalda, voy a evaluar la relación de cada vértebra en su cuello.

I am going to stress your neck in a number of directions to determine whether there is proper movement.
Voy a hacer fuerza sobre su cuello en varias direcciones para determinar si el movimiento es correcto.

I am going to feel the bones and muscles of your neck.
Voy a sentir los huesos y músculos de su cuello.

Thoracic spine
Espina torácica

I am going to place my hands around your rib cage. Breathe out all the way, and then take a very deep breath in.
Voy a colocar mis manos alrededor su caja costal. Exhale completamente y luego inhale profundamente.

Raise your arms up over your head. Bend sideways to the left. Now to the right. Does this produce pain?
Levante sus brazos sobre su cabeza. Dóblese hacia el lado izquierdo. Ahora, dóblese hacia el lado derecho. ¿Esto le produce dolor?

As I palpate your pulse, tip your head back and turn it toward me.
Mientras palpo su pulso, incline su cabeza hacia atrás y vírela hacia mí.

As I palpate your pulse, raise your arm straight out to the side slowly.
Mientras palpo su pulso, levante su brazo hacia los lados lentamente.

As I palpate your pulse, tip your head down as I pull your arm backward.
Mientras palpo su pulso, incline su cabeza hacia abajo mientras yo halo su brazo hacia atrás.

Raise your arms above your head and open and close your fingers and thumbs quickly.
Levante sus brazos sobre su cabeza y abra y cierre los dedos rápidamente.

With you lying face down, I will evaluate the relationship of each vertebra in your mid-back.
Con usted acostado boca arriba, evaluaré la relación de cada vértebra en su espalda media.

With you sitting, I am going to sit directly behind you and stress each vertebra in your mid-back to determine how they are moving.
Con usted sentado, voy a sentarme detrás de usted y le aplicaré fuerza a cada vértebra en su espalda media para determinar cómo se mueven.

Lumbar spine
Espina lumbar

You'll be asked to assume various positions with stresses applied to your body. Tell me whether they make your pain better or worse or cause no change and the location of any pain that is produced.
Se le pedirá que asuma varias posiciones mientras se le aplican fuerzas a su cuerpo. Dígame si éstas mejoran, empeoran o no causan cambios en su dolor y la localización de cualquier dolor que se produce.

In the *standing position*:
Parado:

Bend forward at the waist to touch your toes.
Dóblese hacia delante en la cintura para tocar sus dedos de los pies.

Bend backward at the waist.
Dóblese hacia atrás en la cintura.

Bend to the right.
Dóblese hacia la derecha.

Bend to the left.
Dóblese hacia la izquierda.

Twist your back to the right.
Tuerza su espalda hacia la derecha.

Twist your back to the left.
Tuerza su espalda hacia la izquierda.

Stand on your toes and walk forward two or three steps.
Párese sobre las puntas de sus pies y camine dos o tres pasos hacia delante.

Stand on your heels and walk forward two or three steps.
Párese sobre los talones de sus pies y camine dos o tres pasos hacia delante.

Stand with your feet comfortably apart and close your eyes. I am going to push you lightly.
Párese con sus pies separados cómodamente y cierre los ojos. Voy a empujarlo suavemente.

In the *seated position:*
Sentado:

Straighten your right leg.
Enderece su pierna derecha.

Straighten your left leg.
Enderece su pierna izquierda.

Straighten both legs.
Enderece ambas piernas.

As I support you, lean forward, turn and tip to the right, then bend backward.
Mientras yo le apoyo, dóblese hacia delante, gire e inclínese hacia la derecha y luego dóblese hacia atrás.

As I support you, lean forward, turn and tip to the left, then bend backward.
Mientras yo le apoyo, dóblese hacia delante, gire e inclínese hacia la izquierda y luego dóblese hacia atrás.

I will now tap your leg muscles with this rubber hammer.
Ahora voy a golpear suavemente los músculos de sus piernas con este martillo de goma.

I am going to touch you lightly on your legs. Tell me if there is a difference in sensation from one side to the other.
Voy a tocarlo suavemente en sus piernas. Dígame si hay alguna diferencia en sensación entre un lado y el otro.

I am going to touch your legs with this pin. Tell me if it feels sharp or dull.
Voy a tocar sus piernas con este alfiler. Dígame si se siente afilado o desafilado.

I am going to scrape the handle of the hammer on the bottom of your foot.
Voy a raspar el mango del martillo en la planta de su pie.

I need to test some leg muscles for strength.
Necesito probar la fuerza de algunos de los músculos de la pierna.

Raise your ankle up and in. I am going to pull it down and out; resist.
Levante su tobillo e inclínelo hacia dentro. Voy a tratar de halarlo hacia abajo y hacia fuera; resístase.

Point your toes down and out. I am going to pull your ankle up and in; resist.
Incline sus pies hacia abajo y hacia fuera. Yo voy a halar su tobillo hacia arriba y hacia dentro; resístase.

Raise your big toe up. I am going to pull it down; resist.
Levante el dedo grande del pie. Voy a halarlo hacia abajo; resístase.

I am going to bend your ankle back quickly.
Voy a doblar su tobillo hacia atrás rápidamente.

Close your eyes, straighten both your arms out to the side, and then touch your nose with your index finger from one hand and then with the index finger from other.
Cierre sus ojos, enderece ambos brazos hacia al lado y luego tóquese la nariz con el dedo índice de una mano y luego con el dedo índice de la otra.

I am going to sit directly behind you and stress each of the vertebrae in your lower back to determine how they are moving.
Voy a sentarme detrás de usted y le aplicaré fuerza a cada vértebra en su espalda baja para determinar cómo se mueven.

In the *supine position (lying face up):*
En *posición supina (acostado boca arriba):*

I am going to raise your leg slowly. Don't help, but tell me if it hurts.
Voy a levantar su pierna lentamente. No me ayude, pero dígame si le duele.

I am going to raise your other leg slowly. Don't help, but tell me if it hurts.
Voy a levantar su otra pierna lentamente. No me ayude, pero dígame si le duele.

I am going to raise both of your legs slowly. Don't help, but tell me if it hurts.
Voy a levantar ambas piernas lentamente. No me ayude, pero dígame si le duele.

As I lower both of your legs, try to hold them off the table.
Mientras bajo ambas piernas, trate de mantenerlas despegadas de la mesa.

Slide to the edge of the table and let your leg hang off. I am going to push the other knee toward your chest.
Deslícese hasta el borde de la mesa y deje que su pierna cuelgue. Voy a empujar su otra pierna hacia su pecho.

Put your foot on the opposite knee. I am going to push on this knee.
Coloque su pie en la rodilla opuesta. Voy a empujar sobre esta rodilla.

In the *prone position (lying face down):*
En *posición tendiente (acostado boca abajo):*

I am going to bend your knee and push your heel to your buttock.
Voy a doblar su rodilla y a empujar su talón hasta su nalga.

I am going to bend your knee and push your heel to the opposite buttock.
Voy a doblar su rodilla y a empujar su talón hasta su nalga opuesta.

I am going to bend your knee and lift up on your leg.
Voy a doblar su rodilla y a levantar su pierna.

I am going to place both my hands over your pelvis and apply pressure.
Voy a colocar mis dos manos sobre su pelvis y le aplicaré presión.

I am going to measure your legs for length.
Voy a medir el largo de sus piernas.

With you lying face down, I will evaluate the relationship of each vertebra in your lower back.
Mientras está acostado boca abajo, evaluaré la relación de cada vértebra en su espalda baja.

NEUROMUSCULOSKELETAL ASSESSMENT: EXTREMITY FOCUS
EVALUACIÓN NEUROMUSCULOESQUELÉTICA: ENFOQUE DE EXTREMIDADES

Many of these tests will attempt to provoke your pain. This will give me information on which bones, joints, and muscles are causing problems for you.
Muchas de estas pruebas intentarán provocarle dolor. Esto me dará información de cuáles huesos, articulaciones y músculos están causándole problemas.

Tell me if anything I do to you hurts and where the pain is exactly.
Dígame si algo de lo que hago le causa dolor y dónde exactamente es el dolor.

Where is your pain?
¿Dónde es su dolor?

Shoulder
Hombro

I need to check the overall range of movement for your shoulder.
Necesito examinar el rango de movimiento total de su hombro.

In the *seated position:*
Sentado:

Let your arm hang down to the side.
Deje que su brazo cuelgue a su lado.

Raise your arm from the side and over your head.
Levante su brazo desde su lado hacia encima de su cabeza.

Raise your arm to the front and over your head.
Levante su brazo para que esté al frente suyo y sobre su cabeza.

Bring your arm behind your back.
Lleve su brazo detrás de su espalda.

Raise your arm straight out to the side and bend your elbow so that the hand is forward. Turn your arm so that your hand points all the way down and then all the way up.
Levante su brazo hacia el lado y doble el codo para que la mano esté hacia delante. Vire su brazo de manera que su mano apunte completamente hacia abajo y luego completamente hacia arriba.

Bring your arm across the front of your body.
Lleve su brazo al frente de su cuerpo.

We need to repeat the same movements now as I resist you.
Necesitamos repetir los mismos movimientos mientras yo le hago resistencia.

Bring your arm behind your back and try to touch the opposite shoulder blade.
Lleve su brazo detrás de su espalda y trate de tocar su omóplato opuesto.

Bring your arm behind your head and try to reach the opposite shoulder blade.
Lleve su brazo detrás de su cabeza y trate de tocar su omóplato opuesto.

Place your hand on the opposite shoulder and raise and lower your elbow.
Coloque su mano en el hombro opuesto y suba y baje su codo.

I am going to raise your arm out to the side slightly and then bring it forward.
Voy a levantar su brazo un poco hacia el lado y luego lo llevaré hacia delante.

I am going to press on your shoulder at various locations. Tell me if there is pain.
Voy a presionar sobre su hombro en varios lugares. Dígame si hay dolor.

I am going to feel the bones and muscles of your shoulder.
Voy a sentir los huesos y músculos de su hombro.

I am going to push on your collarbone (clavicle) to evaluate whether it can go forward, backward, and up and down.
Voy a empujar sobre su clavícula para evaluar si puede moverse hacia delante, hacia atrás y hacia arriba y abajo.

In the *supine position (lying face up):*
En *posición supina (acostado boca arriba)*:

I am going to stress your arm forward, backward, and downward as I twist it in and out.
Voy a hacerle fuerza a su brazo hacia delante, hacia atrás y hacia abajo y a la vez que lo tuerzo hacia dentro y hacia fuera.

Raise your arm straight up to the ceiling. I am going to push it up, down, across your body, and away from your body. Resist each of these movements.
Levante su brazo directamente hacia arriba. Voy empujarlo hacia arriba, abajo, cruzando su cuerpo y hacia fuera de su cuerpo. Resístase a cada uno de estos movimientos.

In the *prone position (lying face down):*
En *posición tendiente (acostado boca abajo)*:

I am going to stress your shoulder blade sideways as I twist it in both directions.
Voy a aplicarle fuerza a su omóplato hacia los lados y torcerlo en ambas direcciones.

Elbow
Codo

I need to check the overall range of movement for your elbow.
Necesito examinar el rango de movimiento total de su codo.

Straighten your elbow completely.
Enderece su codo completamente.

Bend your elbow completely.
Doble su codo completamente.

Bend your elbow so that your forearm is straight forward. Turn your hand palm up. Now turn it palm down.
Doble su codo de manera que su antebrazo esté hacia delante. Vire su mano con la palma hacia arriba. Ahora vírela con la palma hacia abajo.

We need to repeat the same movements now as I resist you.
Necesitamos repetir los mismos movimientos mientras yo le hago resistencia.

Make a fist and bend your wrist back. I am going to pull down on your hand; resist.
Haga un puño y doble su muñeca hacia atrás. Voy a halar su mano hacia abajo; resístase.

Bend your elbow so that your forearm is straight forward; turn your hand palm up. I am going to push your hand down; resist.
Doble su codo de manera que su antebrazo esté hacia delante; vire su mano con la palma hacia arriba. Voy a empujar su mano hacia abajo; resístase.

I am going to push against your elbow from each side.
Voy a empujar contra su codo desde cada lado.

Make a fist. Bend your elbow and your wrist back. I am going to pull down on your hand and straighten your elbow; resist.
Haga un puño. Doble su codo y muñeca hacia atrás. Voy a halar su mano hacia abajo y enderezar su codo; resístase.

I am going to tap over parts of your elbow with this rubber hammer. Tell me if you have any sensations.
Voy a golpear suavemente sobre partes de su codo con este martillo de goma. Dígame si tiene alguna sensación.

I am going to stress your elbow in a number of directions to determine if there is proper movement.
Voy a aplicarle fuerza a su codo en varias direcciones para determinar si el movimiento es correcto.

I am going to feel the bones and muscles of your elbow.
Voy a sentir los huesos y músculos de su codo.

Wrist and hand
Muñeca y mano

I need to check the overall range of movement of your wrist and hand.
Necesito examinar el rango de movimiento total de su muñeca y mano.

Move your wrist up and down.
Mueva su muñeca hacia arriba y hacia abajo.

Move your wrist sideways (back and forth).
Mueva su muñeca hacia ambos lados.

Move your fingers up and down.
Mueva sus dedos hacia arriba y hacia abajo.

Curl your fingers tightly and open them up.
Doble sus dedos fuertemente y ábralos.

Spread your fingers apart and bring them together.
Separe sus dedos y luego únalos.

Move your thumb around.
Mueva su dedo pulgar.

We need to repeat the same movements now as I resist you.
Necesitamos repetir los mismos movimientos mientras yo le hago resistencia.

I am going to squeeze your wrist.
Voy a apretar su muñeca.

Touch your thumb to your little finger. I am going to pull them apart; resist.
Toque su dedo meñique con su dedo pulgar. Voy a halarlos para separarlos; resístase.

Make a fist with your thumb inside the fingers. I am going to pull your wrist sideways; resist.
Haga un puño con el dedo pulgar dentro del puño. Voy a halar su muñeca de lado a lado; resístase.

Hold this piece of paper between two fingers as I pull it; resist.
Aguante este pedazo de papel entre dos dedos mientras yo lo halo; resístase.

Put the palms of your hands together and push (praying hands).
Una las palmas de sus manos (manos de oración) y empuje.

Put the backs of your hands together and push.
Una las partes de atrás de sus manos y empuje.

Squeeze this instrument.
Apriete este instrumento.

I am going to tap over parts of your wrist and hand with this rubber hammer. Tell me if you have any sensations.
Voy a golpear suavemente sobre partes de su muñeca y mano con este martillo de goma. Dígame si tiene alguna sensación.

I am going to stress your wrist and hand in a number of directions to determine if there is proper movement.
Voy a hacer fuerza sobre su muñeca y mano en varias direcciones para determinar si el movimiento es correcto.

I am going to feel the bones and muscles of your wrist and hand.
Voy a sentir los huesos y músculos de su muñeca y mano.

Hip
Cadera

I need to check the overall range of movement of your hip.
Necesito examinar el rango de movimiento total de su cadera.

In the *standing position:*
Parado:

Raise your knee to your chest as if you are marching.
Levante su rodilla hasta el pecho como si estuviese marchando.

Swing your thigh backward as far as you can.
Columpie su muslo hacia atrás tan lejos como pueda.

Swing your leg out sideways as far as you can.
Columpie su pierna hacia los lados tan lejos como pueda.

Swing this leg across your other leg as far as you can.
Columpie esta pierna sobre la otra pierna tan lejos como sea posible.

We need to repeat the same movements now as I resist you.
Necesitamos repetir los mismos movimientos mientras yo le hago resistencia.

In the *supine position (lying face up):*
En *posición supina (acostado boca arriba):*

Twist/turn your hip and leg in.
Tuerza/gire su cadera y pierna hacia dentro.

Twist/turn your hip and leg out.
Tuerza/gire su cadera y pierna hacia fuera.

We need to repeat the same movements now as I resist you.
Necesitamos repetir los mismos movimientos mientras yo le hago resistencia.

Put your foot on the opposite knee. I am going to push on this knee.
Ponga su pie sobre la rodilla opuesta. Voy a empujar sobre esta rodilla.

I am going to raise your leg and lightly strike your heel with my fist.
Voy a subir su pierna y golpear suavemente la planta de su pie con mi puño.

Grasp your knee and pull it to your chest.
Agarre su rodilla y hálela hasta su pecho.

I am going to stress your hip in a number of directions to determine whether there is proper movement.
Voy a hacer fuerza sobre su cadera en varias direcciones para determinar si el movimiento es correcto.

I am going to feel the bones and muscles of your hip.
Voy a sentir los huesos y músculos de su cadera.

Knee
Rodilla

I need to check the overall range of movement of your knee.
Necesito examinar el rango de movimiento total de su rodilla.

In the *prone position (lying face down):*
En *posición tendiente (acostado boca abajo):*

Bend your knee to bring your heel as close to your buttock as possible.
Doble sus rodillas para llevar su talón tan cerca de su nalga como sea posible.

Straighten your knee completely.
Enderece su rodilla completamente.

I am going to bend your knee, grasp your foot, apply downward pressure, and twist.
Voy a doblar su rodilla, agarrar su pie y aplicar fuerza hacia abajo y torcerlo.

I am going to bend your knee, grasp your foot, apply upward pressure, and twist.
Voy a doblar su rodilla, agarrar su pie y aplicar fuerza hacia arriba y torcerlo.

In the *supine position (lying face up):*
En *posición supina (acostado boca arriba):*

I am going to push against the side of your knee with your leg straight.
Voy a empujar contra un lado de su rodilla con su pierna recta.

I am going to bend your knee slightly and let go, allowing it to straighten completely.
Voy a doblar su rodilla levemente y dejarla ir para que se enderece completamente.

I am going to apply pressure to your kneecap (patella).
Voy a aplicar presión en su rótula.

Bend your knee, putting your foot flat on the table. I am going to push or pull your knee backward or forward.
Doble su rodilla y ponga su pie plano sobre la mesa. Voy a empujar o halar su rodilla hacia delante o hacia atrás.

With your hip straight up and your knee bent, I am going to straighten your leg while pushing sideways on your knee.
Con su cadera recta y su rodilla doblada, voy a enderezar su pierna mientras empujo hacia los lados su rodilla.

I am going to stress your knee in a number of directions to determine whether there is proper movement.
Voy a hacer fuerza sobre su rodilla en varias direcciones para determinar si el movimiento es correcto.

I am going to feel the bones and muscles of your knee.
Voy a sentir los huesos y músculos de su rodilla.

Ankle and foot
Tobillo y pie

I need to check the overall range of movement of your ankle and foot.
Necesito examinar el rango de movimiento total de su tobillo y pie.

Move your ankle up and down.
Mueva su tobillo hacia arriba y hacia abajo.

Move your ankle sideways (back and forth).
Mueva su tobillo de lado a lado.

Move your toes up and down.
Mueva los dedos de los pies hacia arriba y hacia abajo.

We need to repeat the same movements now as I resist you.
Necesitamos repetir los mismos movimientos mientras yo le hago resistencia.

I am going to squeeze your calf while I bend your ankle.
Voy a apretar su pantorrilla mientras doblo su tobillo.

I am going to squeeze your foot.
Voy a apretar su pie.

I am going to tap over parts of your foot and ankle with this rubber hammer. Tell me if you have any sensation.
Voy a golpear suavemente sobre partes de su tobillo y pie con este martillo de goma. Dígame si tiene alguna sensación.

I am going to stress your ankle and foot in a number of directions to determine whether there is proper movement.
Voy a hacer fuerza sobre su tobillo y pie en varias direcciones para determinar si el movimiento es correcto.

I am going to feel the bones and muscles of your ankle and foot.
Voy a sentir los huesos y músculos de su tobillo y pie.

Temporomandibular Joint (Jaw)
Articulación temporomandibular

I need to check the overall range of movement of your jaw.
Necesito examinar el rango de movimiento total de su mandíbula.

Open your mouth completely.
Abra su boca completamente.

Open and close your mouth three times.
Abra y cierre su boca tres veces.

With your mouth slightly open, move your jaw to the left and to the right.
Con su boca un poco abierta, mueva su mandíbula hacia la derecha y la izquierda.

Close your mouth completely and bite down.
Cierre su boca completamente y muerda.

As I touch your jaw, open and close it three times.
Mientras toco su mandíbula, abra y cierre su boca tres veces.

I am going to place my fingers in your ears. Open and close your mouth three times.
Voy a poner mis dedos en sus oídos. Abra y cierre su boca tres veces.

I need to feel two muscles inside your mouth.
Necesito sentir dos músculos dentro de su boca.

I will use a rubber glove on my hands for protection.
Voy a usar guantes de goma en mis manos para protección.

Try to keep your tongue away from my finger.
Trate de mover su lengua lejos de mi dedo.

I am going to stress your jaw in a number of directions to determine whether there is proper movement.
Voy a hacer fuerza sobre su mandíbula en varias direcciones para determinar si el movimiento es correcto.

I am going to feel the bones and muscles of your jaw.
Voy a sentir los huesos y músculos de su mandíbula.

RADIOGRAPHS (X-RAYS)
RADIOGRAFÍAS (LAS PLACAS)

Radiographs (x-rays) can be helpful as a diagnostic tool.
Las radiografías (las placas) pueden ser útiles como una herramienta de diagnóstico.

Radiographs (x-rays) can provide information about diseases, fractures, and normal and abnormal structural alignment.

Las radiografías (las placas) pueden proveer información acerca de enfermedades, fracturas y alineación estructural normal o anormal.

Radiographs (x-rays) can detect problems not visible during a regular exam.

Las radiografías (las placas) pueden detectar problemas que no son visibles durante un examen regular.

Have you had radiographs (x-rays) taken recently?

¿Le han tomado radiografías (placas) recientemente?

When did have your last radiographs (x-rays) taken?

¿Cuándo fueron tomadas sus últimas radiografías (placas)?

What radiographs (x-rays) were taken?

¿Qué radiografías (placas) se tomaron?

Can you have your radiographs (x-rays) sent to us?

¿Puede hacer que nos envíen las radiografías (placas)?

We will need your permission to have radiographs (x-rays) sent to us.

Necesitaremos su permiso para que nos envíen las radiografías (placas).

I cannot treat you properly if you refuse to have the radiograph (x-ray) taken.

No puedo tratarle apropiadamente si se niega a tomarse las radiografías (placas).

The radiograph (x-ray film) will help me to see your bones and joints clearly.

La radiografía (la placa) me ayudaría a ver sus huesos y articulaciones claramente.

Is there any chance that you are pregnant?

¿Hay alguna posibilidad de que esté embarazada?

Box 5-5 Body regions for x-ray examination	Cuadro 5-5 Regiones corporales para examen radiográfico
Cervical spine	Espina cervical
Thoracic spine	Espina torácica
Lumbar spine	Espina lumbar
Full spine	Espina completa
Shoulder	Hombro
Elbow	Codo
Wrist and hand	Muñeca y mano
Hip	Cadera
Knee	Rodilla
Ankle and foot	Tobillo y pie
Skull	Cráneo

I need to take radiographs (x-rays) of your ________. (See Box 5-5)
Necesito tomar radiografías (placas) de su ________. (Vea el Cuadro 5-5)

When radiographs (x-rays) are taken, all metal must be removed from the area.
Cuando se toman radiografías (placas), hay que remover todo el metal del área.

I need you to put on this gown while radiographs (x-rays) are being taken.
Necesito que use esta bata mientras le toman las radiografías (placas).

Please put this gown on with the opening in the back.
Por favor póngase esta bata con la abertura hacia atrás.

Remove all of your clothing except your underwear, and put this gown on with the opening in the back.
Quítese toda su ropa, excepto su ropa interior, y póngase esta bata con la abertura hacia atrás.

A gonad shield will be used to protect your reproductive organs.
Se usará un escudo de gónada para proteger sus órganos reproductivos.

Place this gonad shield in your underwear.
Coloque este escudo de gónada dentro de su ropa interior.

Radiographs (x-rays) of your spine will be taken with you standing.
Las radiografías de su espina se tomarán con usted parado.

Radiographs (x-rays) of your ________(see Box 5-5) will be taken with you (standing, sitting, lying face up, lying face down).
Las radiografías de su ________ (vea el Cuadro 5-5) se tomarán con usted (parado, sentado, acostado boca arriba, acostado boca abajo).

I will be taking (1, 2, 3, 4, 5, 6, 7, 8, 9) view(s).
Tomaré (1, 2, 3, 4, 5, 6, 7, 8, 9) vista(s).

Please stand here.
Por favor párese aquí.

I need to measure this area.
Necesito medir esta área.

Take a breath in.
Inhale.

Let your breath out.
Exhale.

Hold very still for the radiograph (x-ray).
Manténgase quieto para la radiografía.

Movement can make the radiograph (x-ray) useless.
El movimiento puede hacer la radiografía inútil.

You will not feel the x-rays (any pain or discomfort) as I take the radiograph (x-ray).
Usted no sentirá los rayos x (ningún dolor o molestia) mientras tomo la radiografía.

You will hear the sounds of the x-ray machine during the exposure.
Usted escuchará los sonidos de la máquina de rayos x durante la exposición.

The radiograph (x-ray film) will be developed shortly.
La radiografía (la placa) será revelada en poco tiempo.

There was a (developing/positioning) error and I need to retake the radiograph (x-ray).
Hubo un error de (revelado/posición) y necesito volver a tomar la radiografía.

I am referring you to an imaging center for ________. (See Box 5-6)
Voy a referirle a un centro de imágenes para ________. (Vea el Cuadro 5-6)

Let's look at your radiographs (x-rays).
Veamos sus radiografías.

Box 5-6 Types of advanced imaging	Cuadro 5-6 Tipos avanzados de creación de imágenes
Magnetic resonance imaging (MRI)	Imágenes por resonancia magnética
Computed tomography (CT) scan	Tomografía computarizada
Bone scan	Imagen del hueso
Diagnostic ultrasound examination	Examinación diagnóstica por ultrasonido
Magnetic resonance angiography (MRA)	Angiografía por resonancia magnética

This radiograph (x-ray) of you is from front to back.
Esta radiografía es de usted desde el frente.

This radiograph (x-ray) of you is from the side.
Esta radiografía es de usted desde el lado.

These are your vertebrae.
Estas son sus vértebras.

This vertebra is not aligning properly.
Esta vértebra no está alineada correctamente.

This vertebra hurt when I pushed on it.
Le dolió esta vértebra cuando la empujé.

This is a degenerative change in your disk.
este es un cambio degenerativo en su disco.

The curve in your cervical spine should be increased/decreased.
La curva en su espina cervical debe reducirse/aumentarse.

The curve in your thoracic spine should be increased/decreased.
La curva en su espina torácica debe reducirse/aumentarse.

The curve in your lumbar spine should be increased/decreased.
La curva en su espina lumbar debe reducirse/aumentarse.

Your pelvis is not level.
Su pelvis no está nivelada.

The segments are not aligned properly.
Los segmentos no están alineados correctamente.

This is an x-ray manifestation of ACE (alternating conditional expectation) subluxation.
Esta es una radiografía de un subdislocamiento ACE (expectativa condicional que alterna).

White areas on the radiograph (x-ray) represent bone.
Las áreas blancas en la radiografía representan los huesos.

Black areas on the radiograph (x-ray) represent air.
Las áreas negras en la radiografía representan aire.

Do you have any questions about your radiographs (x-rays)?
¿Usted tiene cualquier pregunta acerca de sus radiografías?

Part 3
Parte 3

Delivery of Care
Administración de Cuidado

Chapter 6
Treatment

Capítulo 6
Tratamiento

EXPLAINING THE APPROACH TO CARE
EXPLICAR LA ESTRATEGIA DE CUIDADO

Complementary and/or supportive care

Cuidado complementario y/o de apoyo

Nutrition: is the use of foods you eat and food-related products to support the body in a healthy way and may include vitamins and minerals.

Nutrición: es el uso de los alimentos que ingiere y de productos relacionados a alimentos para apoyar al cuerpo en una manera saludable y puede incluir vitaminas y minerales.

Diet: is the way you eat, including the kinds of foods and drinks that you consume as meals and snacks.

Dieta: es la manera en que come, incluyendo los tipos de alimentos y bebidas que consume como comidas y meriendas.

Lifestyle: is the way you live your life including your food, exercise, attitude, and stress level.

Estilo de vida: es la manera en que vive su vida incluyendo alimentos, ejercicio, actitud y nivel de estrés.

Posture: is the way you stand and sit.

Postura: es la manera en que se para y se sienta.

The use of other therapies, complementary and alternative medicine (CAM), are those practices for treatment of the body that include health promotion and disease prevention, which are not routinely taught at U.S. medical schools and are not routinely covered by insurance.

El uso de otras terapias, medicina complementaria y alternativa, son aquellas prácticas para el tratamiento del cuerpo que incluyen la promoción de salud y prevención de enfermedades que no son enseñadas rutinariamente en las escuelas de medicina de Estados Unidos y rutinariamente no son cubiertas por los seguros.

Massage: uses hand treatment (rubbing) of the soft tissues or muscles of the body to influence health.

Masaje: usa tratamiento manual (sobar) de los tejidos blandos o músculos del cuerpo para influenciar la salud.

Traditional Chinese medicine: evaluates the condition of the body through diagnosis by means of inspection, listening, smelling, palpation, and inquiry. Treatment is rendered through the use of herbs and sometimes acupuncture and other means.

Medicina china tradicional: evalúa la condición del cuerpo mediante diagnósticos por medio de inspeccionar, escuchar, oler, palpar y preguntar. El tratamiento se provee mediante el uso de hierbas y a veces acupuntura y otros medios.

Acupuncture: evaluation of the balance of energy (an imbalance produces illness) in the body and treatment through the use of needles placed in areas to influence this balance.

Acupuntura: evaluación del equilibrio de energía (un desequilibrio produce enfermedad) en el cuerpo y tratamiento mediante el uso de agujas colocadas en áreas del cuerpo para influenciar este equilibrio.

Other approaches include homeopathy, osteopathy, herbalism, healing touch, aromatherapy, naturopathic medicine, qigong, ayurvedic medicine, traditional healing (*curanderos*—folk healers/*hueseros*—bone healers).
Otros métodos incluyen homeopatía, osteopatía, herbalismo, toque sanador, aromaterapia, medicina naturopática, qigong, medicina ayurvedic, curación tradicional (curanderos/hueseros).

Equipment used in treating conditions
Equipo usado al tratar condiciones

The table
La mesa

I will use this table to help examine and treat you.
Voy a usar esta mesa para examinarle y tratarle.

This table moves up and down like this.
Esta mesa se mueve hacia arriba y hacia abajo, así.

This movement creates traction.
Este movimiento crea tracción.

The headpiece adjusts to make you comfortable.
La cabecera se ajusta para hacerlo sentir cómodo.

This section of the table drops to make some adjustments easier.
Esta sección de la mesa se baja para facilitar algunos de los ajustes.

Instrument
Instrumento

I will use this instrument to adjust your vertebrae/joints.
Voy a usar este instrumento para ajustar sus vértebras/articulaciones.

This instrument is spring loaded and adjustable.
Este instrumento tiene un resorte y es ajustable.

It works like this.
Funciona así.

This instrument is electrical/mechanical and adjusts your joints and works like this.
Este instrumento es eléctrico/mecánico y ajusta sus articulaciones, y funciona así.

Pelvic bench
Banco pélvico

I will use this bench to help me adjust your vertebrae/joints.
Voy a usar este banco para ayudarme a ajustar sus vértebras/articulaciones.

Please kneel on the bench like this.
Por favor arrodíllese sobre el banco, así.

Traction table
Mesa de tracción

I use this table to stretch areas of your body and slightly separate the joints while I adjust your spine/back.
Voy a usar esta mesa para estirar partes de su cuerpo y separar levemente las articulaciones mientras le ajustó su espina/espalda.

This table has an electric motor to assist with traction.
Esta mesa tiene un motor eléctrico para asistir con la tracción.

Please lie on the table while I turn on the motor to make it move.
Por favor acuéstese sobre la mesa mientras enciendo el motor para hacerla mover.

We will treat you gently and slowly.
Vamos a tratarle cuidadosamente y lentamente.

Please let me know if you have any pain during the treatment.
Por favor déjeme saber si tiene cualquier dolor durante el tratamiento.

Exercise
Ejercicio

You can use free weights of various sizes.
Puede usar pesas de varios tamaños.

You can use manual machines for resistance with various weights, such as a cable weight bench.
Puede usar máquinas manuales para resistencia con varios pesos, tales como un banco de pesas de cable.

You can use electric machines with weight or resistance, such as a treadmill.
Puede usar máquinas eléctricas con peso o resistencia, tales como una trotadora.

You can use exercise machines for flexion, extension, and rotation
Puede usar máquinas de hacer ejercicio para flexión, extensión y rotación.

You can use manual and electric machines, which simulate various positions and movements.
Puede usar máquinas manuales y eléctricas para simular varias posiciones y movimientos.

Box 6-1 Patient prompts	Cuadro 6-1 Ordenes para el paciente
Lie face down	Acuéstese boca abajo
Lie face up	Acuéstese boca arriba
Sit	Siéntese
Stand	Párese
Lie on your side facing me	Acuéstese de lado mirando hacia mí
Other side	Del otro lado
Up	Arriba
Down	Abajo
Relax your head/arm/leg	Relaje su cabeza/brazo/pierna
Inhale deeply	Inhale profundamente
Exhale	Exhale
We are finished	Terminamos

Box 6-2 Simple questions during exam and treatment	Cuadro 6-2 Preguntas simples durante el examen y tratamiento
Do you have pain now?	¿Usted tiene dolor ahora?
Do you have pain here?	¿Usted tiene dolor aquí?
Are you okay?	¿Está bien?
Are you comfortable?	¿Está cómodo?

REPORT OF FINDINGS
INFORME DE HALLAZGOS

I would like to go over your history and examination findings with you.
Me gustaría revisar con usted sus antecedentes y los hallazgos de la examinación.

I am going to explain your exam results and discuss treatment options with you.
Voy a explicarle los resultados de sus exámenes y discutir con usted las opciones de tratamiento.

Please feel free to ask questions.
Por favor siéntase libre de hacer preguntas.

You will be advised of choices for care.
Se le asesorará acerca de sus opciones de cuidado.

To help you understand chiropractic practice, I want to discuss some basic principles with you.
Para ayudarle a entender la práctica quiropráctica, quiero discutir algunos principios básicos con usted.

Disturbances of the nervous system may affect your health.
Los trastornos del sistema nervioso pueden afectar su salud.

Environmental changes and physical stress can unduly irritate the nervous system.
Los cambios ambientales y el estrés físico pueden irritar excesivamente el sistema nervioso.

Disturbances of the nervous system may be caused by derangements of the musculoskeletal system.
Los trastornos del sistema nervioso pueden ser causados por desequilibrios del sistema musculoesquelético.

Restricted movement or joint alignment problems of the spine or extremities may contribute to disturbances in the nervous system.
Los problemas de movimiento restringido o de alineación de articulaciones en la espina o las extremidades pueden contribuir a los trastornos del sistema nervioso.

Chiropractors call this type of joint dysfunction *a subluxation.*
Los quiroprácticos llaman a este tipo de disfunción articular *subdislocamiento.*

We believe that optimal structure and function of the musculoskeletal system can assist the body in maintaining health.
Creemos que la estructura y función óptima del sistema musculoesquelético pueden ayudar al cuerpo a mantenerse saludable.

Back pain conditions are the most common complaints for which clients seek help in the chiropractor's office.
Las condiciones de dolor de espalda son las quejas más comunes para las cuales los clientes buscan ayuda en una oficina de un quiropráctico.

Manipulation is the main therapy, along with the use of physical therapy.
La manipulación es la terapia principal, junto con el uso de terapia física.

According to these findings, there are characteristics of subluxation affecting your spine area.
Según estos hallazgos, hay características de subdislocamiento afectando el área espinal.

I believe that your condition has the potential to respond to manipulative therapy.
Yo creo que su condición tiene el potencial para responder a la terapia de manipulación.

Your history and examination findings suggest a diagnosis of ________. (See Box 7-1)
Su historial y los hallazgos de la examinación sugieren un diagnóstico de ________. (Vea el Cuadro 7-1)

Explaining the Adjustment
Explicar el ajuste

The most significant treatment procedure that I use is the chiropractic adjustment.
El procedimiento de tratamiento más importante que yo uso es el ajuste quiropráctico.

The purpose of the adjustment is to normalize the joint relationships in your spine or extremities.
El propósito del ajuste es normalizar las relaciones articulares en su espina o en las extremidades.

Manipulation changes the mechanics of the joints, and with repetition, establishes correct nerve, muscle, and joint function.
La manipulación cambia la mecánica de las articulaciones, y con repetición, establece la función nerviosa, muscular y articular correcta.

The adjustment is a precise maneuver that should not be painful.
El ajuste es un movimiento preciso que no debería ser doloroso.

The chiropractic adjustment is a gentle, yet dynamic thrust applied to a specific joint.
El ajuste quiropráctico es un empuje suave, pero dinámico, que se aplica a una articulación específica.

Although manipulation involves a sudden thrust with speed, it is over an extremely small range of movement.
Aunque la manipulación consiste de un empujón súbito y con velocidad, el mismo es sobre un rango de movimiento extremadamente corto.

The cracking sound comes from a gas bubble in the joint.
El sonido de crujido proviene de una burbuja de gas que está en la articulación.

Chiropractic adjustments restore proper mechanics to the spine.
Los ajustes quiroprácticos restauran la mecánica apropiada de la espina.

Many adjustments will produce a popping noise.
Muchos de los ajustes producirán un sonido de estallido.

The popping noise is not necessary for the adjustment, but it is sometimes surprising when it occurs.
El sonido de estallido no es necesario para el ajuste, pero es en algunas ocasiones sorprendente cuando ocurre.

The popping noise is very similar to the sound made when you crack your knuckles.
El sonido de estallido es similar al sonido producido al astillarse/sonar los nudillos.

Some of the procedures that I will use don't involve a thrust.
Algunos de los procedimientos que usaré no involucran empujes.

Referrals
Referidos

You need to see a ________ for your condition. (See Box 6-3)
Necesita ver a un ________ para su condición. (Vea el Cuadro 6-3)

Do you have a family doctor?
¿Usted tiene un médico de familia?

Would you like me to make an appointment for you?
¿Le gustaría que le hiciera una cita para usted?

I will refer you to Dr. ________.
Le referiré al Dr. ________.

Your appointment is on ________.
Su cita es el ________.

The doctor you will see is________.
El doctor a quien verá es ________.

The doctor's phone number is________.
El número de teléfono del doctor es ________.

The clinic is located at ________.
La clínica está ubicada en ________.

Your condition may be serious. You need to see a ________ as soon as possible.
Su condición puede ser seria. Necesita ver a un ________ tan pronto como sea posible.

You need to have a CT/MRI scan.
Necesita tener una tomografía computarizada/imagen por resonancia magnética.

Box 6-3 Specialists	Cuadro 6-3 Especialistas
Medical doctor	Médico
Family doctor	Médico de familia
Neurologist	Neurólogo
Physical therapist	Terapeuta físico
Cardiologist	Cardiólogo
Gastroenterologist	Gastroenterólogo
Oncologist	Oncólogo
Eye doctor	Oftalmólogo
Radiologist	Radiólogo
Orthopedic surgeon	Cirujano ortopédico
Dentist	Dentista
Emergency room	Sala de emergencia
Urgent care	Cuidado urgente
Paramedic	Paramédico

Emergencies
Emergencias

Your condition is an emergency. We will call an ambulance.
Su condición es una emergencia. Llamaremos a una ambulancia.

You need to go to the emergency room immediately.
Usted necesita ir a la sala de emergencia inmediatamente.

Stay calm. We will stay with you until the ambulance arrives.
Manténgase calmado. Nos quedaremos con usted hasta que llegue la ambulancia.

Chapter 7
Explaining conditions commonly treated by chiropractors

Capítulo 7
Explicar las condiciones comúnmente tratadas por los quiroprácticos

WHIPLASH
LATIGAZO

Is a *condition* caused by a fast stop such as hitting a car or being hit from the rear.
Es una *condición* causada por una parada súbita tal como al chocar con un auto o al ser chocado por atrás.

***Is an injury* to the cervical spine or neck.**
Es una lesión en la espina cervical o el cuello.

***Involves* stretched and torn tendons and ligaments.**
Involucra estiramiento y desgarre de los tendones y ligamentos.

***Symptoms* include:**
Los *síntomas* incluyen:

sore neck
dolor de cuello

headache
dolor de cabeza

difficulty sleeping
dificultad para dormir

aching in the neck and shoulders
dolor en el cuello y los hombros

Box 7-1 Conditions commonly treated by chiropractors	Cuadro 7-1 Condiciones tratadas comúnmente por quiroprácticos
Whiplash	Latigazo
Low back pain	Dolor en la parte baja de la espalda
Sacro-iliac (SI)/pelvic pain	Dolor sacroilíaco/pélvico
Cervical/neck pain	Dolor cervical/de cuello
Muscle spasm and pain	Espasmos y dolores musculares
Headache	Dolor de cabeza
Degenerative joint pain	Dolor en la articulación degenerativo
Carpal tunnel syndrome	Síndrome del túnel carpal
Nonmusculoskeletal problems	Problemas no musculoesqueléticos

Box 7-2 Whiplash	Cuadro 7-2 Latigazo
Neck injury	Lesión en el cuello
Usually caused by auto accident	Usualmente causado por accidentes de automóviles.
Results in stretched and torn tendons and ligaments	Resulta en estiramiento y desgarre de tendones y ligamentos.
Symptoms include soreness, pain, and dysfunction	Los síntomas incluyen dolor y disfunción.
Exam includes neurological and orthopedic tests and x-ray	Los exámenes incluyen pruebas neurológicas y ortopédicas y radiografías.
Treatment includes chiropractic adjustment, therapy, and rehabilitation	El tratamiento incluye ajustes quiroprácticos, terapia y rehabilitación.
Referral is recommended if improvement is not made.	Se recomienda referir si la mejoría no es suficientemente efectiva.

numbness and tingling in the hands and fingers
adormecimiento y hormigueo en las manos y los dedos

sharp pain in the shoulders and arms
dolor agudo en los hombros y brazos

vision problems
problemas en la vista

problems with concentration
problemas de concentración

***Evaluation/examination* includes:**
La *evaluación/examinación* incluye:

neurological and orthopedic testing
examinación neurológica y ortopédica

palpation
palpar

x-ray examination of the area
examinación radiográfica del área

***Treatment* includes chiropractic adjustment and rehabilitation, as well as changes in personal habits.**
El *tratamiento* incluye ajuste quiropráctico y rehabilitación, asi como cambios en los hábitos personales.

***Therapy* may include the use of electrical/nonelectrical devices.**
La *terapia* puede incluir el uso de aparatos eléctricos/no eléctricos.

***Rehabilitation* includes exercises designed specifically to increase flexibility and strength in the neck.**
La *rehabilitación* incluye ejercicios diseñados específicamente para aumentar la flexibilidad y la fuerza en el cuello.

Referral **for further evaluation with CT scan or MRI may be necessary if treatment does not help within a reasonable amount of time.**
Puede ser necesario *referirle* para evaluación adicional con tomografía computarizada o con imágenes por resonancia magnética si el tratamiento no le ayuda dentro de un tiempo razonable.

LOW BACK PAIN
DOLOR EN LA PARTE BAJA DE LA ESPALDA

Is *a condition* of pain in the low part of the spine near the waist.
Es *una condición* de dolor en la parte baja de la columna cerca de la cintura.

The pain:
El dolor:

Box 7-3 Low back pain	Cuadro 7-3 Dolor en la parte baja de la espalda
Pain is felt in the lower part of the back.	El dolor es sentido en la parte baja de la espalda.
Pain may have several causes.	El dolor puede tener varias causas.
Exam includes neurological and orthopedic testing and x-ray.	Los exámenes incluyen pruebas neurológicas y ortopédicas y radiografías.
Treatment includes chiropractic adjustment, therapy, and rehabilitation.	El tratamiento incluye ajustes quiroprácticos, terapia y rehabilitación.
Referral is recommended if improvement is not made.	Se recomienda referir si la mejoría no es suficientemente efectiva.

may be from a disk (cartilage pad between vertebrae) injury in the lumbar spine (low back).
puede ser debido a una lesión en un disco (almohadilla de cartílago entre las vértebras) en la columna lumbar (parte baja de la espalda).

may be from strained muscles, ligaments, or tendons in the area.
puede ser debido a músculos, ligamentos o tendones estirados en el área.

may run down part of a leg (usually the back of the leg) to the feet and toes.
puede extenderse a una parte de una pierna (generalmente la parte de atrás de la pierna) a los pies y dedos de los pies.

may cause the person to lean to one side during the early symptoms (do you lean away from the pain or toward the pain?).
puede causar que la persona se incline hacia un lado durante la fase temprana de los síntomas. ¿Usted se inclina hacia el dolor o hacia el lado contrario?

***Evaluation/examination* includes:**
La *evaluación/examinación* incluye:

palpation
palpar

neurological and orthopedic testing
examinación neurológica y ortopédica

x-ray examination of the area
examinación radiográfica del área

***Treatment* includes:**
El tratamiento incluye:

chiropractic adjustments to the area
ajustes quiroprácticos al área.

muscle massage (deep or superficial)
masajes musculares (profundo o superficial)

rehabilitation
rehabilitación

education in correct lifting
educación acerca del levantamiento correcto

education in nutrition
educación en nutrición

modification of negative personal habits (e.g., use of tobacco, alcohol, and drugs)
modificación de los hábitos personales negativos (por ejemplo, uso de tabaco, alcohol y drogas)

***Therapy* may include the use of electrical/nonelectrical devices.**
La *terapia* puede incluir el uso de aparatos eléctricos/no eléctricos.

***Rehabilitation* involves exercise to increase strength and motion.**
La rehabilitación incluye ejercicios para aumentar la fuerza y el movimiento.

***Referral* for further evaluation including CT scan or MRI may be necessary if chiropractic treatment does not help within a reasonable amount of time.**
Puede ser necesario *referirle* para evaluación adicional con tomografía computarizada o con imágenes por resonancia magnética si el tratamiento quiropráctico no le ayuda dentro de un tiempo razonable.

Box 7-4 Sacroiliac/ pelvic pain	Cuadro 7-4 Dolor sacroilíaco/pélvico
Pain is usually caused by a misalignment in the sacroiliac (SI) joints or pelvis.	Generalmente el dolor es causado por desalineación de las articulaciones sacroilíacas o pélvicas.
Symptoms include pain in the pelvis, but no leg pain.	Los síntomas incluyen dolor en la pelvis, pero no en la pierna.
Exam includes palpation, motion, and x-ray.	El examen incluye palpar, movimiento y radiografías.
Treatment includes chiropractic adjustments, therapy, and rehabilitation.	El tratamiento incluye ajustes quiroprácticos, terapia y rehabilitación.
Referral is recommended if improvement is not made.	Se recomienda referir si la mejoría no es suficientemente efectiva.

SACROILIAC/PELVIC PAIN
DOLOR SACROILÍACO/PÉLVICO

***Causes* of sacroiliac (SI)/pelvic pain include misalignment of the pelvis or sacroiliac joints. Such pain may also originate from an organ in the body.**
Las *causas* del dolor sacroilíaco/pélvico incluyen la desalineación de las articulaciones pélvicas o sacroilíacas. Tal dolor también puede originarse desde un órgano en el cuerpo.

***Located* in the SI area, small joints between the pelvis and the sacrum, the base of the spine.**
Está *localizado* en el área sacroilíaca, pequeñas articulaciones entre la pelvis y el sacro, la base de la espina.

***Resulting* from a misalignment of the joints and stress on the muscles.**
Resulta de una desalineación de las articulaciones y estrés en los músculos.

***Symptoms* include pain over the area of the misalignment but not running down the leg.**
Los *síntomas* incluyen dolor sobre el área de la desalineación pero no se extiende a la pierna.

***Evaluation/examination* of the problem includes:**
La *evaluación/examinación* del problema incluye:

palpation (feeling with the hand) of the area of the pain
palpar (sentir con la mano) el área del dolor

movement or motion of the SI joints
movimiento de las articulaciones sacroilíacas

x-ray examination of the area
examinación radiográfica del área

***Treatment* includes chiropractic adjustments of the joints and massage of the muscles involved.**
El *tratamiento* incluye ajustes quiroprácticos de las articulaciones y masajes musculares.

***Rehabilitation* involves increasing strength and motion.**
La *rehabilitación* incluye ejercicios para aumentar la fuerza y el movimiento.

***Therapy* may include the use of electrical/nonelectrical devices.**
La *terapia* puede incluir el uso de aparatos eléctricos/no eléctricos.

***Referral* for further evaluation may be necessary if chiropractic treatment does not help within a reasonable amount of time.**
Puede ser necesario *referirle* para evaluación adicional si el tratamiento quiropráctico no le ayuda dentro de un tiempo razonable.

CERVICAL/NECK PAIN
DOLOR CERVICAL/DE CUELLO

May have *several causes* including acute trauma. It may be chronic or have a gradual onset over a long period.
Pueden haber *varias causas* incluyendo trauma agudo, el cual puede ser crónico o comenzar lentamente a través de un largo periodo de tiempo.

***Symptoms* include:**
Los *síntomas* incluyen:

sharp or dull pain in the back of the neck or on the right or left side
dolor agudo o sordo en la parte de atrás del cuello o en el lado izquierdo o derecho

numbness and tingling in the arm, hand, or fingers
adormecimiento y hormigueo en el brazo, la mano o los dedos

burning sensation in the arm
sensación ardiente (de ardor) en el brazo

loss of muscle strength in the arm and hand
pérdida de fuerza muscular en el brazo y la mano

pain, possibly located in and caused by muscles in the neck and shoulders
dolor, posiblemente localizado y causado por los músculos del cuello y los hombros

***Evaluation/examination* of the problem includes:**
La *evaluación/examinación* del problema incluye:

palpation of the joints and muscles of the painful area of the neck
palpar las articulaciones y los músculos en el área adolorida del cuello

neurological and orthopedic testing
evaluación neurológica y ortopédica

testing movement/motion in the neck
evaluación del movimiento del cuello

x-ray examination of the area involved
examinación radiográfica del área afectada

***Treatment* includes chiropractic adjustments of the joints and massage of the involved muscles.**
El *tratamiento* incluye ajustes quiroprácticos de las articulaciones y masajes musculares.

***Therapy* may include the use of electrical/nonelectrical devices.**
La *terapia* puede incluir el uso de aparatos eléctricos/no eléctricos.

***Rehabilitation* of the area to increase strength and motion may involve:**
La *rehabilitación* del área para aumentar fortaleza y movimiento puede incluir:

exercise
ejercicio

posture correction
corrección de postura

lifestyle changes
cambios en el estilo de vida

MUSCLE SPASM AND PAIN
ESPASMOS Y DOLORES MUSCULARES

Have several *causes* including acute trauma. Muscle spasm and pain may also be chronic or have a gradual onset over a long period.
Tienen varias *causas* incluyendo trauma agudo. Los espasmos y dolores musculares pueden ser crónicos o comenzar lentamente a través de un largo periodo de tiempo.

***Symptoms* include (Do you have...?):**
Los *síntomas* incluyen (¿Usted tiene . . .?):

sharp or dull pain in the neck
dolor agudo o sordo en el cuello

sharp or dull pain in the shoulder
dolor agudo o sordo en el hombro

sharp or dull pain in the arm
dolor agudo o sordo en el brazo

sharp or dull pain in the back
dolor agudo o sordo en la espalda

sharp or dull pain in the buttocks
dolor agudo o sordo en las nalgas

sharp or dull pain in the leg
dolor agudo o sordo en la pierna

***Pain may be* (Is your pain ...?):**
El *dolor puede ser* (¿Su dolor es . . .?):

spread out
esparcido

located in a specific area
localizado en un área específica

dull
sordo

aching
doloroso

***Evaluation/examination* includes palpation of the area and testing of the adjacent body joints.**
La *evaluación/examinación* incluye palpar el área y examinar las articulaciones circundantes.

***Treatment* includes:**
El *tratamiento* incluye:

cold when pain is acute
frío cuando el dolores es agudo

heat when pain is chronic
calor cuando el dolor es crónico

both heat and cold in long-standing cases
calor y frío en los casos prolongados

deep massage of muscles
masajes profundos de los músculos

chiropractic adjustments of surrounding bone joints
ajustes quiroprácticos de las articulaciones circundantes

***Therapy* may include the use of electrical/nonelectrical devices.**
La *terapia* puede incluir el uso de aparatos eléctricos/no eléctricos.

***X-ray* examination may be performed if treatment does not produce needed improvement.**
Se pueden tomar *radiografías* si el tratamiento no produce las mejorías necesarias.

***Referral* for additional examination may be necessary if improvement is not sufficient.**
Puede ser necesario *referirle* para evaluación adicional si el tratamiento no le ayuda dentro de un tiempo razonable.

HEADACHE
DOLOR DE CABEZA

Causes are:
Las *causas son:*

vascular, neurological, and physiological
vasculares, neurológicas y fisiológicas

***Symptoms* include pain located in (Where is the pain? Is the pain in/on/or ...?):**
Los *síntomas* incluyen dolor en (¿Dónde está el dolor? ¿El dolor está en/o ...?):

the front of the head
el frente de la cabeza

the back of the head
la parte de atrás de la cabeza

the sides of the head
los lados de la cabeza

deep inside the head
profundo en la cabeza

behind the eyes
detrás de los ojos

***Pain characteristics* include (Is the/there pain...?):**
Las *características del dolor* incluyen (¿El dolor es . . .?):

dull
sordo

sharp
agudo

aching pain
doloroso

throbbing pain with possible nausea and vomiting
dolor palpitante posiblemente con náuseas y vómitos

pain with blurred vision
dolor con visión borrosa

pain with dizziness
dolor con mareos

***Evaluation/examination* includes a detailed health history including the following questions about the characteristics of the individual's headache:**
La *evaluación/examinación* incluye un historial detallado incluyendo las siguientes preguntas acerca de las características del dolor de cabeza de la persona:

Where is the headache and is it on one side of the head only?
¿Dónde está el dolor de cabeza y si está es un solo lado de la cabeza?

How long have you had the headache?
¿Cuánto tiempo lleva con el dolor de cabeza?

Do you wake with the pain?
¿Se despierta con el dolor?

Do you have pain at the end of the day?
¿Tiene el dolor al final del día?

Do you have many headaches connected to each other—a cluster?
¿Padece de muchos dolores de cabeza conectados unos a otro?

Is the pain focused on some part of the head?
¿El dolor está enfocado en una parte de la cabeza?

***Neurological* testing may be required to find the cause.**
Puede requerirse examinación *neurológica* para encontrar la causa.

***X-ray* examination is important to see and understand the structure of the neck.**
La examinación *radiográfica* es importante para ver y entender la estructura del cuello.

***Ruling out certain diagnoses* is also important because there may be a more serious cause for the headache.**
También es importante *descartar ciertos diagnósticos* porque pueden haber causas más serias que producen el dolor de cabeza.

***Treatment* may include:**
El *tratamiento* puede incluir:

chiropractic adjustments of the neck and upper back
ajustes quiroprácticos del cuello y la parte alta de la espalda

deep massage of neck and shoulder muscles
masajes profundos de los músculos del cuello y los hombros

electrical therapy of areas in the neck and shoulders
terapia eléctrica de las áreas del cuello y los hombros

use of heat or cold packs on adjacent areas
uso de compresas frías o calientes en las áreas adyacentes

exercise associated with the treatment
ejercicio asociado con el tratamiento

***Therapy* may include the use of electrical/nonelectrical devices.**
La *terapia* puede incluir el uso de aparatos eléctricos/no eléctricos.

If treatment does not improve the condition within a reasonable amount of time, then *referral* for further testing and/or treatment is appropriate.
Si el tratamiento no le ayuda dentro de un período de tiempo razonable, puede ser necesario *referirle* para evaluación adicional y/o tratamiento.

DEGENERATIVE JOINT PAIN
DOLOR EN LA ARTICULACIÓN DEGENERATIVO

***Caused* by deterioration of the joint structure, sometimes with an accumulation of calcium or extra bone in or near the joint.**
Es *causado* por el deterioro de la estructura de la articulación, algunas veces con la acumulación de calcio o hueso adicional en o alrededor de la articulación.

***Symptoms* include pain in the affected area.**
Los *síntomas* incluyen dolor en el área afectada.

***Pain characteristics* include:**
Las *características de dolor* incluyen:

deep aching pain
dolor profundo

burning pain
dolor ardiente

throbbing pain
dolor punzante

sharp pain
dolor agudo

Have you had episodes of arthritis-type joint pain before?
¿Usted ha tenido episodios de algún dolor parecido a la artritis anteriormente?

***Areas affected* by this pain include (Have you had pain in the ...?):**
Las *áreas afectadas* por este dolor incluyen (¿Usted ha tenido este dolor en . . .?

neck
el cuello

spine
la espina

joints of the arms, wrists, and fingers
las articulaciones de los brazos, las muñecas y los dedos

joints of the hips, knees, feet, and toes
las articulaciones de las caderas, las rodillas, los pies y los dedos de los pies

Sports participation (In what sports have you ever participated...? And for how long?):
Participación deportiva (¿Qué deportes ha prácticado? ¿Y por cuánto tiempo?)

Have you played soccer?
¿Usted ha practicado fútbol?

Have you played football (American with contact)?
¿Usted ha practicado fútbol americano con contacto?

Have you played tennis?
¿Usted ha jugado tenis?

Have you played basketball?
¿Usted ha jugado baloncesto?

Have you played golf?
¿Usted ha jugado golf?

Have you been a runner?
¿Usted ha sido un corredor?

Other?
¿Otro?

Present sports participation (In what sports do you participate now? Any of those I just mentioned?)
Participación deportiva actual (¿Qué deportes practica ahora? ¿Algunos de los que ya mencioné?)

***Evaluation/examination* includes:**
La *evaluación/examinación* incluye:

palpation of the painful area
palpar el área adolorida

testing of movement of the painful area
examinación del movimiento del área adolorida

x-ray examination of the painful area
examinación radiográfica del área adolorida

orthopedic and neurological testing of the painful area
evaluación ortopédica y neurológica del área adolorida

***Treatment* includes:**
El *tratamiento* incluye:

adjustment and mobilization of the affected joints
ajustes y movilización de las articulaciones afectadas

massage of the surrounding muscles and other soft tissues
masaje de los músculos y otros tejidos blandos adyacentes

moderate exercise within pain tolerance to increase flexibility and strength
ejercicio moderado dentro de las tolerancias del dolor para aumentar la fortaleza y flexibilidad

***Therapy* may include the use of electrical/nonelectrical devices.**
La *terapia* puede incluir el uso de aparatos eléctricos/no eléctricos.

***Referral* is recommended if the treatment is not sufficiently effective in controlling the pain.**
Se recomienda un *referido* si el tratamiento no es suficientemente efectivo en controlar el dolor.

***Pain may be resistive* to treatment, and finding an effective treatment may require perseverance by patient and doctor.**
El *dolor puede ser resistente* al tratamiento y el encontrar un tratamiento efectivo puede requerir perseverancia por parte del paciente y el doctor.

CARPAL TUNNEL SYNDROME
SÍNDROME DEL TÚNEL CARPAL

Defined as a *complex of symptoms* in the hand and fingers caused by pressure on the median nerve at the wrist.
Se define como un *complejo de síntomas* en las manos y los dedos de las manos causado por presión sobre el nervio central en la muñeca.

Generally, the *cause* is some repetitive activity or age degeneration. However, the cause may be unknown.
Generalmente, la *causa* es algún tipo de actividad repetitiva o degeneración por edad. Sin embargo, la causa puede ser desconocida.

***Symptoms* of the condition include:**
Los *síntomas* de la condición incluyen:

numbness and tingling of fingers 3, 4, and 5 (Do you have numbness/tingling of fingers 3, 4, and 5?)
adormecimiento y hormigueo en los dedos 3, 4 y 5 (¿Usted tiene adormecimiento/hormigueo de los dedos 3, 4 y 5?)

nighttime waking with numb hand/fingers (Do you have nighttime waking with numbness in your hand/fingers?)
despertarse en medio de la noche con la mano/los dedos de las manos adormecidos. (¿Usted se despierta en medio de la noche con la mano/los dedos de las manos adormecidos?)

loss of hand grip strength (Do you have loss of grip strength?)
pérdida de fuerza de agarre en las manos (¿Usted ha perdido su fuerza de agarre?)

loss of feeling in the fingers (Do you have loss of feeling in your fingers?)
pérdida de sensación en los dedos de las manos (¿Usted ha perdido sensación en los dedos de las manos?)

muscle wasting in hand (Do you have muscle wasting in your hand in the thenar muscle near the thumb?)
desgaste del músculo en la mano (¿Usted tiene desgaste muscular en su mano en el músculo de la palma de la mano cerca del dedo pulgar?)

Examination/evaluation includes:
La *evaluación/examinación* incluye:

***Health history of activities* of work and leisure over time.**
Historial de salud de actividades de trabajo y placer a través del tiempo.

What kind of work physical activity have you done for the last 10 years?
¿Qué tipo de actividad física de trabajo ha hecho en los últimos 10 años?

What hobbies have you had?
¿Qué pasatiempos ha tenido?

Have you given birth in the last 10 years (if female)?
¿Usted ha tenido hijos en los últimos 10 años (si es mujer)?

Examination of orthopedic and neurological signs include:
La examinación de los signos ortopédicos y neurológicos incluyen:

sensitivity of hand and fingers (Do you have normal sensitivity of hand and fingers to touch?)
sensibilidad en las manos y los dedos de las manos (¿Usted tiene sensibilidad al tacto normal en las manos y los dedos de las manos?)

grip strength of hand (Do you have normal strength of hand in response to testing?)
fuerza de agarre en la mano (¿Usted tiene una fuerza normal en la mano en respuesta a la evaluación?)

pinch strength of fingers (Do you have normal pinch grip strength in fingers?)
fuerza de pinchar en los dedos de las manos (¿Usted tiene una fuerza de agarre de pinza normal en los dedos de las manos?)

point sensitivity of fingers (Do you have normal point sensitivity in your fingers?)
sensibilidad en la punta de los dedos (¿Usted tiene una sensibilidad en la punta de los dedos de las manos?)

***Treatment* includes:**
El *tratamiento* incluye:

adjustment and mobilization of the affected joints of the hand, wrist, and elbow
ajuste y movilización de las articulaciones de la mano, la muñeca y el codo

adjustment of the cervical and upper thoracic spine
ajuste de la espina cervical y torácica superior

massage of the surrounding muscles and other soft tissues, especially in the forearm and the affected hand
masaje de los músculos y otros tejidos blandos circundantes, especialmente en el antebrazo y mano afectada

exercise of the wrist and muscles in the forearm to counter stress from overactivity
ejercicio de la muñeca y los músculos del antebrazo para contrarrestar el estrés de la sobreactividad

rest from stressful activity for the affected wrist and arm to allow for healing
descanso de actividades estresantes para la muñeca y el brazo afectado para permitir curación

***Therapy* may include the use of electrical/nonelectrical devices.**
La *terapia* puede incluir el uso de aparatos eléctricos/no eléctricos.

***Rehabilitation* includes flexibility and strengthening exercises, especially exercises opposing normal activities (i.e., exercise in the opposite direction from normal use).**
La *rehabilitación* incluye ejercicios de flexibilidad y fortalecimiento, especialmente ejercicios opuestos a la actividad normal (por ejemplo, ejercicios en dirección opuesta al uso normal).

***Referral* is recommended if the treatment is not sufficiently effective in managing pain and numbness and tingling.**
Se recomienda *referir si* el tratamiento no es suficientemente efectivo para combatir el dolor, adormecimiento y hormigueo.

***Other treatment* may include surgery on the affected wrist if chiropractic treatment is not effective (surgery of the wrist/hand to expand space for the median nerve).**
Otros tratamientos pueden incluir cirugía en la muñeca afectada si el tratamiento quiropráctico no es efectivo (cirugía en la muñeca/mano para expandir el espacio para el nervio central).

DEGENERATIVE JOINT PAIN
DOLOR EN LA ARTICULACIÓN DEGENERATIVO

***Causes* include acute injuries to extremity with a joint and/or soft tissue effect.**
Las *causas* incluyen lesiones agudas a las extremidades con un efecto en la articulación y/o tejido blando.

***Located* in the extremities of the body including (Do you have pain in the...):**
Está *localizado* en las extremidades del cuerpo incluyendo (¿Usted tiene dolor en . . .?):

shoulder
el hombro

elbow
el codo

wrist/hand/fingers
la muñeca/la mano/los dedos de las manos

hip
la cadera

knee
la rodilla

ankle
el tobillo

feet/toes
los pies/los dedos de los pies

***Resulting* from a possible misalignment of the joints and stress on the muscles in the extremities**
Resulta de una posible desalineación de las articulaciones y tensión en los músculos en las extremidades.

***Symptoms* in the area of the strain/sprain include:**
Los *síntomas* en el área de torcedura/dislocadura incluyen:

tenderness and soreness over the area
sensibilidad y dolor sobre el área

possible swelling over the area
inflamación posible sobre el área

***Evaluation/examination* of the problem includes:**
La *evaluación/examinación* del problema incluye:

palpation (feeling with the hand) of the area of the pain
palpar (sentir con la mano) el área del dolor

movement of the SI joints
movimiento de las articulaciones sacroilíacas

x-ray examination of the area
examinación radiográfica del área

***Treatment* includes chiropractic adjustments of the joints and massage of the muscles involved.**
El *tratamiento* incluye ajustes quiroprácticos de las articulaciones y masajes musculares.

***Therapy* may include the use of electrical/nonelectrical devices.**
La *terapia* puede incluir el uso de aparatos eléctricos/no eléctricos.

***Rehabilitation* includes increasing strength/motion.**
La *rehabilitación* incluye aumentar la fortaleza/el movimiento.

***Referral* for further evaluation may be necessary if chiropractic treatment is not helpful within a reasonable amount of time.**
Puede ser necesario *referirle* para evaluación adicional si el tratamiento quiropráctico no le ayuda dentro de un tiempo razonable.

SACROILIAC JOINT PROBLEMS
PROBLEMAS DE ARTICULACIÓN SACROILÍACOS

***Causes* include misalignment of the pelvis or SI joints. Problems may also originate from disease in or damage to an internal organ.**
Las *causas* incluyen desalineación de las articulaciones pélvicas o sacroilíacas. Los problemas también pueden originarse en enfermedad o daño a un órgano interno.

***Located* in the SI area, small joints between the pelvis and the sacrum, the base of the spine.**
Está *localizado* en el área sacroilíaca, pequeñas articulaciones entre la pelvis y el sacro, la base de la espina.

***Resulting* from a misalignment of the joints and stress on the muscles.**
Resulta de una desalineación de las articulaciones y tensión en los músculos.

***Symptoms* include pain over the area of the misalignment but not running down the leg.**
Los *síntomas* incluyen dolor sobre el área de la desalineación pero no se extiende a la pierna.

***Evaluation/examination* of the problem includes:**
La *evaluación/examinación* del problema incluye:

> **palpation (feeling with the hand) of the area of the pain**
> palpar (sentir con la mano) el área del dolor

movement of the SI joints
movimiento de las articulaciones sacroilíacas

x-ray examination of the area
examinación radiográfica del área

***Treatment* includes chiropractic adjustments of the joints and massage of the muscles involved.**
El *tratamiento* incluye ajustes quiroprácticos de las articulaciones y masajes musculares.

***Therapy* may include the use of electrical/nonelectrical devices.**
La *terapia* puede incluir el uso de aparatos eléctricos/no eléctricos.

***Rehabilitation* includes increasing strength/motion.**
La *rehabilitación* incluye aumentar la fortaleza/el movimiento.

***Referral* for further evaluation may be necessary if chiropractic treatment is not helpful within a reasonable amount of time.**
Puede ser necesario *referirle* para evaluación adicional si el tratamiento quiropráctico no le ayuda dentro de un tiempo razonable.

NONMUSCULOSKELETAL PROBLEMS
PROBLEMAS NO MUSCULOESQUELÉTICOS

Defined as organic problems in the body and concerned with an organ system.
Se define como problemas orgánicos en el cuerpo y atañe con un sistema de órgano.

The *cause* could be any kind of disease or damage, ranging from an upset stomach to cancer of the liver or some other organ.
La *causa* puede ser cualquier tipo de enfermedad o daño, que varía desde problemas estomacales hasta cáncer del hígado o algún otro órgano.

***Symptoms* of the condition range from mild pain to complete dysfunction.**

Los *síntomas* de la condición varían desde dolor leve hasta disfunción total.

***Examination/evaluation* includes consideration of all organs in the body that may be related to the problem and may include laboratory and other tests to determine the cause and the extent of the condition.**

La *evaluación/examinación* incluye consideración de todos los órganos del cuerpo que puedan estar relacionados al problema y puede incluir análisis de laboratorio y otras pruebas para determinar la causa y la extensión de la condición.

***Chiropractic treatment* includes adjustment of the bony joints and soft tissue of the body in areas affected. The effect is through the neuromusculoskeletal system (nerves/muscles and bones) of the body.**

El *tratamiento quiropráctico* incluye ajuste de las articulaciones óseas y del tejido blando del cuerpo en las áreas afectadas. El efecto es a través del sistema neuromusculoesquelético (nervios/músculos) del cuerpo.

***Recovery* from the problem requires rest and time to heal.**

La *recuperación* para el problema requiere descanso y tiempo para curarse.

***Referral* is recommended if the treatment is not sufficiently effective in correcting the primary problem within a reasonable amount of time.**

Se recomienda *referir* si el tratamiento no es suficientemente efectivo en corregir el problema principal dentro de un tiempo razonable.

***Other treatment* may include medications and sometimes surgery.**

Otro tratamiento puede incluir medicamentos y en algunas ocasiones cirugía.

English-to-Spanish Terminology

Terminología de Inglés a Español

Days of the Week	Los Días de la Semana
Monday	lunes
Tuesday	martes
Wednesday	miércoles
Thursday	jueves
Friday	viernes
Saturday	sábado
Sunday	domingo

Months	Los Meses
January	enero
February	febrero
March	marzo
April	abril
May	mayo
June	junio
July	julio
August	agosto
September	septiembre
October	octubre
November	noviembre
December	diciembre

Ordinal Numbers	Numerales Ordinales
first	primero/a
second	segundo/a
third	tercero/a
fourth	cuarto/a
fifth	quinto/a
sixth	sexto/a
seventh	séptimo/a
eighth	octavo/a
ninth	noveno/a
tenth	décimo/a

Cardinal Numbers		Números Cardinales
0	zero	cero
1	one	uno/a
2	two	dos
3	three	tres
4	four	cuatro
5	five	cinco
6	six	seis
7	seven	siete
8	eight	ocho
9	nine	nueve
10	ten	diez
11	eleven	once
12	twelve	doce
13	thirteen	trece
14	fourteen	catorce
15	fifteen	quince
16	sixteen	dieciséis
17	seventeen	diecisiete
18	eighteen	dieciocho
19	nineteen	diecinueve
20	twenty	veinte
21	twenty-one	veintiuno
22	twenty-two	veintidós
23	twenty-three	veintitrés
24	twenty-four	veinticuatro
25	twenty-five	veinticinco
26	twenty-six	veintiséis
27	twenty-seven	veintisiete
28	twenty-eight	veintiocho
29	twenty-nine	veintinueve
30	thirty	treinta
40	forty	cuarenta
50	fifty	cincuenta
60	sixty	sesenta
70	seventy	setenta
80	eighty	ochenta
90	ninety	noventa
100	one hundred	cien (ciento)
101	one hundred one	ciento uno
102	one hundred two	ciento dos

103	one hundred three	ciento tres
104	one hundred four	ciento cuatro
105	one hundred five	ciento cinco
106	one hundred six	ciento seis
107	one hundred seven	ciento siete
108	one hundred eight	ciento ocho
109	one hundred nine	ciento nueve
110	one hundred ten	ciento diez
200	two hundred	doscientos
300	three hundred	trescientos
400	four hundred	cuatrocientos
500	five hundred	quinientos
600	six hundred	seiscientos
700	seven hundred	setecientos
800	eight hundred	ochocientos
900	nine hundred	novecientos
1000	one thousand	mil
1991	one thousand nine hundred ninety-one	mil novecientos noventa y uno
2001	two thousand one	dos mil y uno

Interrogative	Palabras Interrogativas
How?	¿Cómo?
How far?	¿A qué distancia?
How often?	¿Con qué frecuencia?
How much?	¿Cuánto?
How many?	¿Cuántos?
How long?	¿Cuánto tiempo?
How many times?	¿Cuántas veces?
What?	¿Qué?
What else?	¿Qué más?
What for?	¿Para qué?
When?	¿Cuándo?
Where?	¿Dónde?
From where?	¿De dónde?
To where?	¿Adónde?
Which?	¿Cuál?
Which (ones)?	¿Cuáles?
Who?	¿Quién?
To whom?	¿A quién?
Whose?	¿De quién?
Why?	¿Por qué?

Expressions of Time	Expresiones de Tiempo
year	el año
month	el mes
week	la semana
day	el día
hour	la hora
minute	el minuto
second	el segundo
today	hoy
tomorrow	mañana
day after tomorrow	pasado mañana
yesterday	ayer
day before yesterday	anteayer
tonight	esta noche
last night	anoche
tomorrow morning	mañana por la mañana
tomorrow afternoon	mañana por la tarde
tomorrow evening	mañana por la noche
every morning	cada mañana, todas las mañanas
every afternoon	cada tarde, todas las tardes
every evening	cada noche, todas las noches
every night	cada noche
in the morning	por la mañana
in the afternoon	por la tarde
in the evening	por la noche
at night	en la noche
all morning	toda la mañana
all afternoon	toda la tarde
all night	toda la noche
two days ago	hace dos días
three weeks ago	hace tres semanas
six years ago	hace seis años
always	siempre
never	nunca
sometimes	algunas veces
from time to time	de vez en cuando
now	ahora
right now	ahora mismo
before	antes
after	después
later	más tarde

next week	la semana próxima
until	hasta

Clothing / La Ropa

bathing suit	el traje de baño
bathrobe	la bata (de baño)
belt	el cinturón
blouse	la blusa
blue jeans	los levis, los jeans, los vaqueros
boot	la bota
brassiere	el sostén, los portabustos
button	el botón
cap	la gorra
coat	el abrigo
collar	el cuello
corset	el corsé
diaper	el pañal
dress	el vestido
hat	el sombrero
heel	el tacón
(low) heels	los tacones bajos
high heels	los tacones altos
hose	las medias
jacket	la chaqueta
light weight (light clothes)	ligero (la ropa ligera)
oxfords	los zapatos bajos
panties	los pantaletas, las pantis
pants	los pantalones
sandals	las sandalias
scarf	la bufanda
shirt	la camisa
t-shirt	la camiseta
shoe	el zapato
shorts (men's)	los calzones, los calzoncillos
skirt	la falda, la pollera
sleeve	la manga
long	larga
short	corta
slipper	la zapatilla, la chancleta
sneakers	los zapatos de goma
sock(s)	el calcetín, los calcetines

stockings	las medias
suit	el traje
sweater	el suéter
tie	la corbata
trousers	los pantalones
underpants	los calzoncillos
underwear	la ropa interior, la ropa íntima
(under)shirt	la camiseta
vest	el chaleco

Family Members (Relatives) / Miembros de la Familia (Parientes)

aunt	la tía
brother	el hermano
brother-in-law	el cuñado
children	los hijos, los niños
cousin	el/la primo/a
daughter	la hija
daughter-in-law	la nuera
father	el padre, el papá
father-in-law	el suegro
grandfather	el abuelo
grandmother	la abuela
husband	el esposo, el marido, "el viejo" (slang)
in-laws	los suegros
mother	la madre, la mamá
mother-in-law	la suegra
nephew	el sobrino
niece	la sobrina
parents	los padres
sister	la hermana
sister-in-law	la cuñada
son	el hijo
son-in-law	el yerno
uncle	el tío
wife	la esposa, la mujer, "la vieja" (slang)

TIME ON THE CLOCK

[To tell time in Spanish use the verb *ser* + *la(s)* and the number.]

What time is it?
¿Qué hora es?

It is seven o'clock.
Son las siete.

It is one o'clock.
Es la una.

It is eight o'clock.
Son las ocho.

It is two o'clock.
Son las dos.

It is nine o'clock.
Son las nueve.

It is three o'clock.
Son las tres.

It is ten o'clock.
Son las diez.

It is four o'clock.
Son las cuatro.

It is eleven o'clock.
Son las once.

It is five o'clock.
Son las cinco.

It is twelve o'clock.
Son las doce.

It is six o'clock.
Son las seis.
[Use "media" for "30" or half past the hour.]

It is 3:30.
Son las tres y media.
AM = de la mañana
PM = de la tarde (till 6 o'clock)
PM = de la noche (from 6 till midnight)
On the right side of the clock use "y" when expressing minutes:

It is ten after one.
Es la una y diez.

It is two fifteen.
Son las dos y cuarto.

It is three fifteen.
Son las tres y quince.

It is three thirty.
Son las tres y media.
On the left side of the clock use "menos" or "falta(n)"

It is twenty to two.
Son las dos menos veinte.

It is five to eight.
Son las ocho menos cinco.

It is twenty to two.
Faltan veinte para las dos.

It is five to eight.
Faltan cinco para las ocho.

TIME EXPRESSIONS

At what time?
¿A qué hora?

At eight o'clock
A las ocho

At noon
Al mediodía

At midnight
A la medianoche

early
temprano

late
tarde

on time
a tiempo

Colors	**Los Colores**
black	negro/a
blue	azul
bluish	azulado
brown	café, marrón
clear, light (in color tone)	claro/a
dark	oscuro/a
gold	dorado/a
green	verde
grey	gris
orange	anaranjado/a
pale	pálido/a
pink	rosa
purple	púrpura, morado/a
red	rojo, colorado
reddish	rojizo
silver	plateado/a
transparent	transparente
white	blanco/a
yellow	amarillo/a
yellowish	amarillento

The Office	La Oficina
administration	la administración
assistant	el/la asistente
bathroom	el baño, el servicio
cashier	el/la cajero/a
chair	la silla
door/doorway	la puerta/la entrada
e-mail	el correo electrónico
entrance	la entrada
exam (room/room)	el (salón/cuarto) de examen
exam record	el expediente
exit	la salida
fax	el fax
front desk	el mostrador
hallway	el pasillo
insurance	el seguro
insurance company	la compañía de seguro
insurance form	el formulario del seguro
laboratory	el laboratorio
mail	el correo
paperwork	el papeleo
public phone	el teléfono público
receptionist	el/la recepcionista
specialist	el/la especialista
telephone	el teléfono
reception room	la sala de espera, la recepción
treatment room	el cuarto de tratamiento

General Health	La Salud General
allergy	la alergia
asthma	el asma
arthritis	la artritis
blood sugar	el azúcar de la sangre, la glucosa
breathing problems	los problemas respiratorios
bruise	el moretón
cancer	el cáncer
cold	el catarro, el resfriado
contagious	contagioso/a
diabetes	la diabetes
drug sensitivity	la sensibilidad al medicamento

fever	la fiebre
freckle	la peca
flu	la gripe
headache	el dolor de la cabeza
heart problems	los problemas cardíacos
HIV positive	el VIH positivo
high blood pressure	la presión sanguínea alta, la tensión alta
joint replacement	reemplazo de la coyuntura
measles	el sarampión
pregnant	embarazada, esperando familia, en estado
rheumatic fever	la fiebre reumática
scarlet fever	la fiebre escarlatina
thyroid problem	los problemas de la tiroides
wart	la verruga

Diseases/Conditions	**Enfermedades/ Condiciones**
blindness	la ceguera
burn	la quemadura
cut	la cortadura
infection	la infección
inflammation	la inflamación
injury	la lesión
mucous	mucoso
scar	la cicatriz
stitches	los puntos
surgery	la cirugía
trauma	el golpe
wound	la herida

Symptoms	**Los Síntomas**
ache	duele
burn	quema
cough	tos
dizzy	mareado/a
ear ache	dolor de oído
gradual	gradual
irritation	la irritación
itch	la comezón, el picazón
pain	el dolor

redness	el enrojecimiento
sharp pain	el dolor agudo
sinus pain	el dolor nasal
sudden	repentino/a, a súbito
swelling	la hinchazón
tired	cansado

Medications	**Medicamentos**
antibiotic	el antibiótico
capsules	las cápsulas
daily	diariamente
drops	las gotas
pharmacy	la farmacia
pills	las pastillas
shake well	agite bien
tablets	las tabletas

CHIROPRACTIC TERMS

Biomechanics	la biomecánica
Blood cuff	el baumanómetro
Carpal tunnel syndrome (CTS)	el síndrome del túnel carpal
Chiropractic lesion	la lesión quiropráctica
Chiropractic manipulation/ adjustment	la manipulación/el ajuste quiropráctico
Chiropractic table	la mesa quiropráctica
Cold therapy	la terapia fría
Comprehensive medical history	el historial médico exhaustivo
Compression fracture	la fractura por compresión
Computer screen	la pantalla de la computadora
Condyle	el cóndilo
Confidentiality	la discreción
Congenital disorder	el desorden congénito
Degenerative joint pain	el dolor degenerativo en la articulación
Dislocate	dislocar
Distraction	la distracción
Electrical therapy	la terapia eléctrica
Exercise	el ejercicio
Extremity	la extremidad
Fall	la caída

Film	la película
Fracture	la fractura
Gait	el porte
Headache	el dolor de cabeza
Heat therapy	la terapia caliente
Jaw	la mandíbula
Joint	la articulación
Lateral	lateral
Limitations	las limitaciones
Lips	los labios
Low back pain	el dolor en la parte baja de la espalda
Musculoskeletal problems	los problemas musculoesqueléticos
Massage	el masaje
Muscle spasm	el espasmo muscular
Neurological testing	el análisis neurológico
Nutrition	la nutrición
Orthopedic testing	el examen ortopédico
Oto-ophthalmoscope	el oto-oftalmoscopio
Pain	el dolor
Palpation pelvic bench	el banco de palpación pélvica
Play	jugar
Posture	la postura
Rehabilitation	la rehabilitación
Rubber hammer	el martillo de goma
Side posture table	la mesa de postura lateral
Slip	resbalón
Soft tissue	el tejido blando
Sprain	torcer
Step	el paso
Stethoscope	el estetoscopio
Stool	el taburete
Strain	la torcedura
Subluxation	la subluxación vertebral
Supports	los apoyos
Teeth	los dientes
Temporomandibular disorder	el desorden temporomandibular
Temporomandibular joint	la coyuntura temporomandibular
Therapeutic exercise	el ejercicio terapéutico

Therapy	la terapia
Thermometer	el termómetro
Tongue	la lengua
Tooth	el diente
Traction	la tracción
Treatment	el tratamiento
Trip	tropezar
Tuning fork	el diapasón
Vital signs	los signos vitales
Whiplash	latigazo
Work	el trabajo
X-ray	la radiografía

Spanish-to-English Terminology

Terminología de Español a Inglés

A

abril	April
la abuela	grandmother
el abuelo	grandfather
la administración	administration
¿adónde?	to where?
agite bien	shake well
agosto	August
ahora	now
ahora mismo	right now
a la medianoche	at midnight
a las ocho	at eight o'clock
algunas veces	sometimes
al mediodía	at noon
la presión sanguínea alta	high blood pressure
amarillento/a	yellowish
el análisis neurológico	neurological testing
anoche	last night
anteayer	day before yesterday
los anteojos	glasses
antes	before
el antibiótico	antibiotic
¿a qué distancia?	how far?
¿a qué hora?	at what time?
el año	year
el próximo año	next year
los apoyos	supports
¿a quién?	to whom?
la articulación	joint
la artritis	arthritis

a tiempo	on time
el aumento	power
ayer	yesterday
el/la ayudante, el/la asistente	assistant
el azúcar de la sangre	blood sugar
azul	blue
azulado/a	bluish

B

el banco de palpación pélvica	palpation pelvic bench
el baño	bathroom
el baumanómetro	blood cuff
la biomecánica	biomechanics
blanco/a	white

C

cada mañana	every morning
cada noche	every night
cada tarde	every afternoon
café	brown
el/la cajero/a	cashier
la caída	fall
cansado/a	tired
las cápsulas	capsules
el catarro	cold
catorce	fourteen
la ceguera	blindness
la ceja	eyebrow
cero	zero
la cicatriz	scar
cien	one hundred
ciento	one hundred
ciento cinco	one hundred five
ciento cuatro	one hundred four
ciento diez	one hundred ten
ciento dos	one hundred two
ciento nueve	one hundred nine
ciento ocho	one hundred eight
ciento seis	one hundred six
ciento siete	one hundred seven

ciento tres	one hundred three
ciento uno	one hundred one
cinco	five
cincuenta	fifty
la cirugía	surgery
claro/a	clear, light (in color tone)
colorado/a	red
la columna	spine
la comezón	itch
¿cómo?	how?
el cóndilo	condyle
¿con qué frecuencia?	how often?
contagioso/a	contagious
la coyuntura temporomandibular	temporomandibular joint
¿cuál?	which?
¿cuáles?	which (ones)?
¿cuándo?	when?
¿cuántas veces?	how many times?
¿cuánto?	how much?
¿cuántos?	how many?
¿cuánto tiempo?	how long?
cuarenta	forty
cuarto/a	fourth
cuatro	four
cuatrocientos	four hundred
la cuñada	sister-in-law
el cuñado	brother-in-law

D

décimo/a	tenth
¿de dónde?	from where?
el defecto	defect
de la mañana	A.M. (in the morning)
de la noche	P.M. (from 6 till midnight)
de la tarde	P.M. (till 6 o'clock)
¿de quién?	whose?
de repente	suddenly
el desorden congénito	congenital disorder
el desorden temporomandibular	temporomandibular disorder
después	after

de vez en cuando	from time to time
el día	day
la diabetes	diabetes
día de la semana	day of the week
el diapasón	tuning fork
diariamente	daily
diciembre	December
diecinueve	nineteen
dieciocho	eighteen
dieciséis	sixteen
diecisiete	seventeen
el diente	tooth
los dientes	teeth
diez	ten
la discreción	confidentiality
torcer	sprain
doce	twelve
el dolor	pain
el dolor degenerativo en la articulación	degenerative joint pain
el dolor de la cabeza	headache
el dolor en la parte baja de la espalda	low back pain
domingo	Sunday
¿donde?	where?
dorado/a	gold (in color tone)
dos	two
doscientos	two hundred
dos mil y uno	two thousand one

E

el ejercicio	exercise
el ejercicio terapéutico	therapeutic exercise
embarazada	pregnant
enero	January
la enfermedad	disease
la entrada	entrance
es la una y diez	it is ten after one
el espasmo muscular	muscle spasm
esperando familia	pregnant
la esposa	wife
el esposo	husband

esta noche	tonight
en estado	pregnant
el estetoscopio	stethoscope
el examen ortopédico	orthopedic testing
el expediente	exam record
la extremidad	extremity

F

la falta de atención	distraction
faltan cinco para las ocho	it is five to eight
faltan veinte para las dos	it is twenty to two
la farmacia	pharmacy
febrero	February
la fiebre	fever
la fractura	fracture
la fractura por compresión	compression fracture

G

el globo del ojo	eyeball
el golpe	trauma
la gorra	cap
gradual	gradual
la gripe	flu
gris	grey

H

hace dos días	two days ago
hace seis años	six years ago
hace tres semanas	three weeks ago
hasta	until
la herida	wound
la hermana	sister
el hermano	brother
la hija	daughter
el hijo	son
los hijos	children
el historial médico exhaustivo	comprehensive medical history
la hora	hour
hoy	today

I

la infección	infection
la inflamación	inflammation
la irritación	irritation

J

jueves	Thursday
jugar	play
julio	July
junio	June

L

lateral	lateral
latigazo	whiplash
los labios	lips
el laboratorio	laboratory
la lengua	tongue
la lesión	injury
la lesión quiropráctica	chiropractic lesion
las limitaciones	limitations
lunes	Monday

M

la madre	mother
la mandíbula	jaw
la manipulación/el ajuste quiropráctico	chiropractic manipulation/adjustment
mañana	tomorrow
mañana por la mañana	tomorrow morning
mañana por la noche	tomorrow evening
mañana por la tarde	tomorrow afternoon
la mamá	mother
mareado/a	dizzy
el marido	husband
martes	Tuesday
el martillo de goma	rubber hammer
marzo	March
el masaje	massage

más tarde	later
mayo	May
los medicamentos	medications
el mes	month
la mesa de postura lateral	side posture table
la mesa quiropráctica	chiropractic table
miércoles	Wednesday
mil	one thousand
mil novecientos noventa y uno	one thousand nine hundred ninety-one
el minuto	minute
el moco	mucous (n.)
morado/a	purple
el moretón/la hematoma	bruise
mucoso	mucous (adj.)
la mujer	wife
los músculos	muscles

N

negro/a	black
los niños	children
novecientos	nine hundred
noveno/a	ninth
noventa	ninety
noviembre	November
la nuera	daughter-in-law
nueve	nine
el número	number
nunca	never
la nutrición	nutrition

O

ochenta	eighty
ocho	eight
ochocientos	eight hundred
octavo/a	eighth
octubre	October
la oficina	office
el ojo	eye
once	eleven

oscuro/a	dark
el oto-oftalmoscopio	oto-ophthalmoscope

P

el padre	father
los padres	parents
pálido/a	pale (in color tone)
la pantalla de la computadora	computer screen
el pañal	diaper
el papá	father
¿para qué?	what for?
los parientes	relatives
pasado mañana	day after tomorrow
el pasillo	hallway
el paso	step
las pastillas	pills
la película	film
la piel	skin
plateado/a	silver (in color tone)
por la mañana	in the morning
por la noche	in the evening
por la tarde	in the afternoon
¿por qué?	why?
el porte	gait
la postura	posture
primero/a	first
el/la primo/a	cousin
los problemas cardíacos	heart problems
los problemas del tiroides	thyroid problems
los problemas musculoesqueléticos	musculoskeletal problems
púrpura/morado/a	purple

Q

¿qué?	what?
¿qué hora es?	what time is it?
la quemadura	burn
¿qué más?	what else?
¿quién?	who?
quince	fifteen
quinientos	five hundred
quinto/a	fifth

R

la radiografía	radiograph, x-ray
el/la recepcionista	receptionist
la receta	prescription
la rehabilitación	rehabilitation
resbalón	slip
el resfriado	cold
rojizo/a	reddish
rojo/a	red
la ropa	clothing
rosa	pink

S

sábado	Saturday
la salida	exit
el (salón/cuarto) de examen	exam room
el salón de espera	waiting room
la salud	health
el segundo	second (of time)
segundo/a	second
seis	six
seiscientos	six hundred
la semana	week
la próxima semana	next week
septiembre	September
séptimo/a	seventh
el servicio	bathroom
sesenta	sixty
setecientos	seven hundred
setenta	seventy
sexto/a	sixth
siempre	always
siete	seven
los signos vitales	vital signs
la silla	chair
el síndrome del túnel carpal	carpal tunnel syndrome (CTS)
los síntomas	symptoms
la sobrina	niece
el sobrino	nephew
el sombrero	hat

son las cinco	it is five o'clock
son las cuatro	it is four o'clock
son las diez	it is ten o'clock
son las doce	it is twelve o'clock
son las dos	it is two o'clock
son las dos menos veinte	it is twenty to two
son las dos y cuarto	it is a quarter past two
son las nueve	it is nine o'clock
son las ocho	it is eight o'clock
son las ocho menos cinco	it is five to eight
son las once	it is eleven o'clock
son las seis	it is six o'clock
son las siete	it is seven o'clock
son las tres	it is three o'clock
son las tres y media	it is three thirty
son las tres y quince	it is three fifteen
la subluxación (vertebral)	subluxation
la suegra	mother-in-law
el suegro	father-in-law
los suegros	in-laws

T

las tabletas	tablets
el taburete	stool
tarde	late
el tejido blando	soft tissue
el teléfono público	public phone
temprano	early
la terapia	therapy
la terapia caliente	heat therapy
la terapia fría	cold therapy
la terapia eléctrica	electrical therapy
tercero/a	third
el termómetro	thermometer
la tía	aunt
el tío	uncle
toda la mañana	all morning
toda la noche	all night
toda la tarde	all afternoon
todas las mañanas	every morning
todas las noches	every evening

todas las tardes	every afternoon
la torcedura	strain
el trabajo	work
la tracción	traction
transparente	transparent
el tratamiento	treatment
trece	thirteen
treinta	thirty
tres	three
trescientos	three hundred
tropezar	trip

U

uno/a	one

V

los vasos sanguíneos	blood vessels
veinte	twenty
veinticinco	twenty-five
veinticuatro	twenty-four
veintidós	twenty-two
veintinueve	twenty-nine
veintiocho	twenty-eight
veintiséis	twenty-six
veintisiete	twenty-seven
veintitrés	twenty-three
veintiuno	twenty-one
verde	green
la verruga	wart
"la vieja"	wife
"el viejo"	husband
viernes	Friday

Y

el yerno	son-in-law

Informal Expressions*

Expressiones Informales

Really? Cool!
¿De veras? !Qué chévere!

Awesome!
¡Qué padre!/¡Excelente!/¡Fabuloso!

My God!
¡Díos mío!

My goodness!
¡Díos mío!

(All right then/Now what)?
¿Y ahora qué?

(All done/Ready to move on)?
¿Ya estuvo?

You didn't notice what happened?
¿No te (das/diste) cuenta?

Don't lose heart. (Don't give up.)
No te dés por vencido.

Don't worry/Don't get upset.
No te agites.

*Modified from Chou B: *Practical Spanish in eyecare*, Boston, 1995, Butterworth-Heinemann.

Index

K

L

M

N

O

P

Índice